Sexual Health and Wellbeing

An Evidence-Based Guide to Desire, Pleasure, and Real-Life Intimacy for All Bodies and Orientations

Lauren Pierce

Legal Disclaimer and Safety Notice

This book provides general educational information about sexual health and wellbeing. It is not medical, psychological, legal, or professional advice. It is not a substitute for diagnosis, treatment, or care from a licensed clinician. Always consult a qualified health professional about your personal situation before applying any information from this book.

Adults only

The content is intended for readers who are 18 years of age or older. If you are under 18, do not use this material.

Consent, safety, and legality

All activities discussed require clear, ongoing, and enthusiastic consent from all participants. The reader is responsible for complying with all applicable laws and age-of-consent rules in their jurisdiction. Do not engage in any activity that causes pain, injury, or distress. Stop immediately if you experience discomfort or if consent is withdrawn.

Health and risk

Sexual activity and use of products can carry physical and emotional risks. If you are pregnant, have a pelvic, cardiovascular, neurological, or mental health condition, or are taking prescription drugs that may affect sexual function, seek individualized guidance from your clinician first. Do not rely on this book in place of emergency care. If you experience severe pain, bleeding, injury, chest pain, shortness of breath, or thoughts of self-harm, call your local emergency number or go to the nearest emergency department.

No guarantee of results

Outcomes vary across individuals. References to tools, products, or websites are provided for convenience only and do not constitute endorsement. Trademarks and brand names remain the property of their respective owners.

Privacy and examples

Any case examples are composites or are used with permission. They are not intended to depict actual persons or to predict individual outcomes.

No professional relationship

Reading this book does not create a doctor-patient, therapist-client, or other professional relationship with the authors or publisher.

Limitation of liability

To the fullest extent permitted by law, the authors and publisher disclaim all liability for any loss, injury, or damages, direct or indirect, that may result from the use of or reliance on this material.

Jurisdiction

The information is written for a general U.S. audience. Readers outside the United States should seek advice from local professionals and follow local laws and standards.

Contents

Chapter 1
Why Sexual Health and Wellbeing Matter

When we talk about health, we usually think of blood pressure, sleep, nutrition, maybe mental balance. Sexuality belongs in that list, because it affects self-esteem, intimacy, and even how safe we feel inside relationships. People who experience ease with sex often describe themselves as more present in their bodies. People who run into obstacles around sex often feel confused, lonely, or convinced that they missed some basic instruction.

In many families and schools, sexual education arrived in pieces. Protect yourself. Avoid pregnancy. Be careful about reputation. Those messages were designed to keep people safe, but they were incomplete. No one explained how desire shows up differently from person to person. No one said that pleasure is a skill. No one warned that stress, caregiving, illness, and grief can mute arousal. So a lot of adults grew up thinking that sex is supposed to be automatic, and if it is not, something is wrong with them.

At the heart of this book is a simple position: sexual response is organized. Slow arousal, intermittent desire, orgasm that requires a certain kind of stimulation, withdrawal after an uncomfortable or frightening experience, all of these are meaningful reactions. Bodies are always responding to context. They pay attention to safety, to stress, to whether touch feels wanted, to what a person has been taught about gender, morality, and worth. Judging the body for doing its job tends to make things worse. Learning how it works tends to make things better.

Consider what happens when sex becomes something you have to perform. A partner wants more than you do. Media tells you that everyone else is having adventurous sex every week. You start monitoring your own arousal and measuring it against a standard that does not come from you. That monitoring creates pressure. Pressure activates the parts of the nervous system that watch for risk. Arousal needs the opposite. It needs time, safety, and a feeling of welcome.

Popular culture does not help. The dominant story of sex is short, symmetrical, and unrealistic. Two people kiss, both become instantly aroused, intercourse happens, both climax. That story is centered on one type of body and one sequence. It almost never shows people who want long, slow external touch. It rarely shows disabled bodies. It does not show the couple who still love each other but spend every night putting kids to bed. It does not show survivors of trauma. When real life looks different, people blame themselves instead of blaming the script that erased them.

A more accurate way to see desire is to look at the two systems in the brain that manage sexual response. One system notices erotic, affectionate, or exciting cues and starts to move toward them. The other scans for reasons to pause, such as pain, fear of pregnancy, lack of privacy, resentment, religious guilt, or simple exhaustion. Some people have very lively approach systems. Others have very sensitive pause systems. Neither pattern is a failure. Trouble starts when life keeps pressing the pause system every day, so desire cannot get traction even if the person likes sex in principle.

Safety sits underneath everything. Real consent is not only a yes. It is a yes that could have been a no. When someone believes that sex is owed, or that saying no will lead to sulking or anger, the body often answers by reducing arousal. Dryness, loss of erection, pelvic floor tension, or checking out mentally are not always dysfunctions. Sometimes they are protective responses. Sexual health requires relational health, which means respect for limits, time to warm up, and the right to change your mind.

Shame can act like a low, constant brake. If you were taught that good people do not enjoy sex too much, or that your body is the source of temptation, or that being desired is dangerous, you may find it hard to relax in erotic situations. Shame says, hide. Sexuality asks, be seen. That conflict can silence desire. Healing in this area does not ask you to reject your values. It asks you to decide which values help you love and be loved as an adult.

There is another pattern that deserves attention. Some people learned to use sex as a tool to keep closeness. They said yes to avoid conflict, to reassure a partner, to reduce their own fear of abandonment. At the beginning this can look generous. Over time it becomes costly. The body stops sending desire because it has not been listened to. The way forward is not to push for more sex. The way forward is to bring honesty into the bedroom: I want touch but not penetration tonight, or I need repair first, or I need to feel wanted too.

Long relationships change the way desire works. At the start, novelty, uncertainty, and anticipation act like natural accelerators. You think about the person and your body responds. Years later the context is different. You know each other well. There is laundry, work, maybe illness, maybe caregiving, certainly stress. Stress is a strong brake. In this phase desire often becomes responsive instead of spontaneous. It appears after you start, not before. Many people interpret this as loss of attraction. It is usually just a different mode of desire.

Private erotic life belongs in a discussion of health. Masturbation, fantasy, and other forms of solo sex are normal, common, and useful. They help you learn what kind of stimulation works, how long you need, and what kind of mental imagery supports arousal. That knowledge feeds partnered sex because you can describe what you like. Solo sex becomes a problem mainly when it is used to avoid communication or when it hides distress that should be addressed.

Sexual diversity must be included from the beginning. Some people are asexual or only rarely experience sexual attraction. Some people need deep emotional intimacy to want sex. Some value sensual closeness over orgasm. Others experience intense desire at certain points in hormonal cycles and very little the rest of the time. Sexual wellbeing does not require a fixed frequency. It requires that your experience fits your body, your relationships, and your values.

Medical realities also shape erotic life. Hormonal contraception, antidepressants, diabetes, pelvic pain, endometriosis, pregnancy, postpartum changes, perimenopause, menopause, disability, gender-affirming treatments, all can affect arousal, lubrication, erection, or orgasm. Too many people stay silent about this in medical settings because sex still feels like an optional topic. It is not. Sexual comfort is part of health care. You are allowed to ask for options and referrals.

All of these strands meet in one skill: agency. Sexual wellbeing means you can say what kind of sexual life you want, you can talk about it with partners, and you can adapt when life changes. That almost always requires better conversations. A large number of sexual problems are actually communication problems that were never solved. Clear, kind, specific talk calms uncertainty. Calm bodies notice pleasure more easily.

The chapters that follow will unpack desire and arousal, walk through anatomy for different bodies, question cultural and gender scripts, address trauma and healing, include queer and trans experiences, look at porn and digital intimacy, and end with a personal plan you can adjust over time. The goal stays practical: more safety, more choice, more pleasure, more room to be the sexual person your real life can support.

Chapter 2
Your Body, Your Context: How Stress, Safety, and Culture Shape Desire

Human sexual desire is often presented as a built-in drive that should appear on command, always at the same level, almost independent from the circumstances; in real adult lives, though, desire behaves far more like a responsive system that keeps asking, "Am I safe, am I rested, am I respected, am I wanted, do I have privacy, do I have time, do I have permission?", and only when several of those conditions are met does the body decide to move toward pleasure. If those conditions are missing, what you see is not failure but a sensible pause.

Consider the contrast between two very ordinary situations. During a weekend away, when no one is knocking at the bedroom door, when meals are already handled, when there is no laptop in sight and no one expects answers, many people discover that arousal can appear with almost no effort, as if it had been waiting nearby. During a crowded workweek, in a small apartment, with messages arriving, with children awake, with money on the mind, the very same body and the very same relationship can appear almost nonsexual. That difference does not come from personality. It comes from context.

Stress is usually the first element to examine because the nervous system is designed to prioritize protection over reproduction or pleasure. When the brain marks something as urgent, whether that urgency is emotional, financial, social, or physical, it allocates attention and energy to solving that issue, and in doing so it turns down interest in activities that require openness, slowness, and vulnerability. Short bursts of stress can be absorbed and later released. Chronic stress, the kind that stretches across months due to unpaid labor, conflict, health problems, or caregiving, keeps the brake pressed most of the time and leaves very little space for erotic curiosity, no matter how much affection exists in the couple.

Safety works in the opposite direction. A person who knows that their no will be honored, that their body will not be pushed past pain, that requests for slower touch or more warm up will be taken seriously, and that disclosure of past experiences will not be used against them, often discovers a gradual increase in desire simply because the nervous system is no longer occupied with monitoring for danger. In that sense, sexual safety is not an abstract value but a physiological condition that clears cognitive and emotional bandwidth so that pleasure can even register.

Daily life in couples shows this very clearly. Imagine one partner arriving home, moving through cooking, messages from family, homework with children, laundry, and mental planning for tomorrow; by the time the evening is quiet, their body is still in task mode and has not had any transition into sensual attention. If, in the same household, burdens were distributed more fairly, if affectionate touch had appeared already during the day, if screens were away, if there was some decompression together, the invitation to sex later would have landed on a much readier nervous system. The difference is not attraction. It is sequence.

Culture enters even earlier than partners. From childhood onward, people receive rules about what sex is for, who may initiate, how often couples "should" have it, what counts as real sex, and whose pleasure matters the most. A woman socialized to be agreeable may keep suppressing her own arousal patterns in order to maintain harmony, until she no longer remembers what she enjoys. A man socialized to show interest at all times may override tiredness, sadness, or fear, because he has learned that any interruption in desire could be read as weakness. Queer, trans, and gender nonconforming people often have to negotiate sexuality in environments that either ignore their bodies or condemn their practices, so their erotic life may become cautious or portioned out only to very safe contexts. None of this is random. It is learned adaptation.

Religious and family narratives can reinforce those pathways. If you were taught for years that sex is sacred only under very narrow conditions, your body may require more trust and more slowness before it allows high arousal, even if, intellectually, you now believe sex is positive. If you were told that penetration is the central or only valid act, you may overlook the forms of pleasure that actually work best for your body. If, growing up, genitals and pleasure were not named at all, talking about them today may feel childish or embarrassing. That is not a fixed trait in you; it is an absence of rehearsal, and rehearsal can happen in adulthood too.

Another contextual element, often invisible but extremely powerful, is the distribution of emotional and cognitive labor. In many heterosexual homes, one person remembers doctor appointments, school events, pantry levels, social obligations, aging parents, vacation planning, and birthday gifts, while also doing a portion of the physical chores. That permanent planning state keeps the brain oriented toward future tasks and away from present-moment bodily sensation. Because sexual attention is present-focused and body-focused, a chronically planning person will need more time and more deliberate transition to enter an erotic scene. Fairer labor, very concretely, makes more room for sex.

Bodies are shaped not only by tasks and beliefs but also by images. When media keeps presenting a very narrow, young, thin, able, smooth, energetic, always-interested body as the erotic norm, it becomes easy for people with postpartum bellies, surgical scars, mobility differences, weight changes, aging skin, or gender-affirming surgeries to think, "My body should not be looked at," and once that thought is present, the person may dim lights, rush encounters, refuse oral sex, or avoid certain positions. Desire then appears low, although the underlying issue is not desire at all but self-consciousness. Sexual well-being asks that the real body, the one that exists today, be invited into pleasure.

The emotional climate in a relationship is another part of context and is frequently underestimated. Desire rarely emerges in an atmosphere of chronic criticism, contempt, or unresolved hurt, because the body does not want to become vulnerable with someone it is defending against. Conversely, when partners repair after conflict, express appreciation during the day, share laughter, and practice affection on days when sex will not happen, they create warmth, and warmth reduces vigilance. Reduced vigilance is one of the shortest paths to more arousal.

Past harm sits even deeper. People who have lived through coercion, assault, unwanted penetration, persistent pressure, or sex that was consistently painful often develop protective responses such as pelvic floor tension, checking out mentally during touch, sudden loss of lubrication, or a general reduction in desire. Those responses are intelligent. They are the nervous system's way of preventing repetition of harm. Expecting such a system to respond to sex without first restoring safety is unfair. What usually helps is a combination of trauma-informed therapy, medical treatment when pain is present, clear communication with partners, and a pace that is set by the survivor rather than by the couple's habits.

Physiological changes interact with all of this. Hormonal contraception, antidepressants, diabetes, endometriosis, pelvic floor dysfunction, pregnancy, postpartum shifts, perimenopause, menopause, disability, and gender-affirming care can all alter lubrication, erection, and speed of arousal. That does not mean desire is gone forever. It means the old sexual script may no longer fit and must be rewritten with more preparation, more direct stimulation, more lube, more focus on pleasure instead of performance, and sometimes with medical support. Bodies change; context can be updated to match.

A practical way to use this chapter is to name, in plain language, the two columns of your life: on one side whatever tells your body yes (privacy, rest, being desired, affection during the day, tidy spaces, fairness, humor, emotional repair, feeling attractive) and on the other side whatever says not now (pain, fear of pregnancy or STIs, resentment, exhaustion, criticism, religious guilt, too many chores, money anxiety, untreated trauma). Many people try to multiply the yes items while leaving the strongest not now untouched and then wonder why desire has not moved. Often the breakthrough comes from removing or reducing one heavy brake rather than adding ten tiny accelerators.

Communication is what allows context to be shared instead of guessed. A partner cannot start earlier in the evening unless they know that late night is the worst moment for you. They cannot slow down their initiation style unless they understand that your body needs transition time from worker or parent into lover. They cannot help with housework unless they realize that mental load turns off your erotic attention. Sentences such as, "I need to be off duty before I can want you," or, "I want more touch on days we do not have sex," or "I need to know I can stop without consequence," are not rejections; they are instructions for building a better context.

In the next chapter we will go inside the model that explains these patterns in a very concrete way, the dual control model, which describes sexual response as the balance between what activates and what inhibits. Once you can see which elements in your own life are pressing the accelerator and which are holding the brake, you can design conditions that support desire instead of waiting for it to appear in a context that keeps saying no.

Chapter 3
Arousal, Desire, and the Dual Control Model

If the first two chapters hinted that desire is responsive, here is where we make that responsibility visible. Your sexual system is built with two complementary processes. One notices sexually relevant information and prepares the body to engage. The other notices anything that could make sex risky, awkward, painful, or costly, and slows things down. Researchers describe this as the dual control model: an excitation system and an inhibition system, operating together all the time, talking to each other in real time, adjusting to context, history, mood, and meaning.

Think of the excitation system first. This is the part of your brain that pays attention to erotic cues. Those cues can be external, such as a partner you find attractive, affectionate touch, a smell, a certain kind of voice, privacy, a fantasy, a setting that feels luxurious or playful. They can also be internal, such as ovulation, hormonal peaks, memories of good sex, or simply being well rested. When the excitation system receives enough cues, it increases interest, attention, and physiological readiness. This is the part of you that says, yes, this could be good.

Now look at the inhibition system. This part notices anything that could lead to bad outcomes. No lock on the door. A partner who seems angry. Fear of pregnancy. Pain during penetration. A history of shaming comments. A room that is too cold, too cluttered, too public. Worries about performance. Anxiety about smell or appearance. A body that is still on alert from daytime stress. Inhibition is not the enemy of sexuality. It is the guardian of sexuality. It says, yes, but only when we are really safe.

People differ in how sensitive each system is. Some have excitation systems that light up easily and inhibition systems that are relaxed. These are the people who can get aroused quickly, in many settings, with minimal preparation, and who often report spontaneous desire even under stress. Others have excitation systems that need specific conditions and inhibition systems that are very watchful. These are the people who want sex in theory, enjoy it once they start, but do not feel desire coming out of nowhere, especially when life is heavy. Both patterns are normal. Problems begin when someone with a sensitive brake lives in a life that presses that brake all the time.

An important distinction appears here: spontaneous desire and responsive desire. Spontaneous desire is the kind most people see in movies. You are walking through the room, you see your partner, and you want sex. Responsive desire is different. You do not feel much at first. Then there is kissing, touch, a sense of connection, and desire grows in response to that. Responsive desire is very common in long relationships, in people with strong inhibition systems, in people carrying a lot of stress, and in people who need emotional closeness first. Calling responsive desire "low desire" is a misunderstanding. It is a different entry point.

Misunderstandings become painful when partners have different entry points. One person may experience frequent spontaneous desire and read that as evidence of love and attraction. The other may need context and touch before feeling anything and read their own lack of spontaneity as failure. If no one explains that both systems are normal and that responsive desire is widely documented, the couple may create a story where one person is the "sexual" one and the other is deficient. The dual control model dissolves that story. It says, you are both working exactly as designed, but your brakes and accelerators are tuned differently.

In practice, excitation can be increased. People can add cues that their bodies recognize as erotic. That may mean more affectionate touch on nonsexual days, more deliberate flirting, more visual or audio erotic material, more attention to smells and lighting, more privacy, more time between tasks and sex, more sex-positive conversations, more mental rehearsal through fantasy. When the brain receives these signals, it becomes easier for desire to arise. This is why vacations, hotels, and getaways so often correlate with better sex: they offer clusters of excitation cues and remove several inhibitory ones at once.

Inhibition, on the other hand, can be reduced. You can close the door. You can get reliable contraception. You can address pain through pelvic floor therapy or medical treatment. You can clean the room so it stops distracting you. You can ask a partner to change their initiation style. You can seek trauma-informed therapy if old experiences are intruding. You can agree on a signal that stops the encounter at any time. Each removed brake makes the accelerator more effective, even if the accelerator itself has not changed.

What people often try first is to push the accelerator harder. Buy lingerie. Watch porn together. Schedule sex. Send suggestive messages. None of that is bad. It simply has limited effect when the brake underneath is something heavy, like resentment, exhaustion, fear, or pain. The dual control model suggests a different order. Before adding arousing stimuli, remove or soften the biggest inhibitors. Many times, when the brake is lighter, ordinary touch becomes arousing again without extra effort.

This model also helps explain why trauma, shame, or chronic criticism have such a strong effect on sexuality. Those experiences teach the inhibition system to be vigilant. The system learns, sex can hurt me, sex can expose me, sex can make me judged, sex can make me powerless. Once that learning is in place, the body becomes slow, not because it dislikes pleasure, but because it is busy protecting the self. In those cases, excitation cues must be especially safe, predictable, and affirming. The person may need more reassurance, more time, more control over pacing, and more positive experiences before the inhibition system trusts again.

Another area where the model is useful is sexual pain. If penetration has been painful, or if the pelvic floor is tense, the inhibition system is doing exactly what it should do by reducing arousal or lubrication. The solution is not to convince yourself to want sex more. The solution is to listen to the inhibition, address the pain, involve competent medical and physiotherapy professionals, and then reintroduce sexual touch in ways that do not hurt. Once the body learns, this is comfortable, inhibition relaxes.

Men and women, as groups, sometimes present different patterns, not because of biology alone, but because of socialization. Many women live with more chronic stress, more learned vigilance, more body shame, and more fear of being judged. That builds stronger brakes. Many men are taught to interpret arousal as proof of masculinity, so they focus on excitation and overlook inhibition until it becomes very strong, for example through performance anxiety. Understanding that everyone has both systems makes it easier to speak about difficulties without assigning blame to the person or to the gender.

This is also the space where fantasy belongs. Erotic fantasy is a way of feeding the excitation system directly with mental cues. It is private, controllable, and adjustable. For people with responsive desire, fantasy can be a bridge into sexual attention. For people with strong brakes, fantasy can help identify which elements feel unsafe. If a person can become aroused in fantasy but not with a partner, the difference is probably inhibition connected to the partner or to the context, not lack of desire in general.

Communication between partners becomes more precise once they have this language. Instead of, "You never want sex," the conversation can become, "Your accelerator seems to need more warm up than mine," or, "My brake is very sensitive to stress, so if we want more sex we have to reduce what presses it," or, "I feel desire after we start, so I need you to initiate even if I look neutral at the beginning." That kind of talk removes moral judgment and replaces it with problem-solving.

The dual control model also encourages curiosity about individual cues. Some people are turned on by novelty, others by familiarity. Some by verbal affirmation, others by a partner's scent. Some by lingerie, others by a clean, quiet room. Some by explicit erotic media, others by romantic narratives. Some by power exchange, others by total equality. Identifying your own excitatory cues gives you tools. Identifying your own inhibitory cues gives you control. You can then build situations that stack the first and reduce the second.

In the next chapter we will look at pleasure and at how to learn what actually feels good in your body, because arousal and desire are only the beginning of sexual experience. For now, keep the model close: your accelerator is working, your brake is working, and much of sexual wellbeing is learning when to add and when to subtract.

Chapter 4
Pleasure: Learning What Feels Good and Why

A lot of people grow up with the quiet assumption that pleasure should arrive ready-made, that you touch the right place and the body simply knows what to do, and if it does not then you must have been born without the so-called "sexual instinct." That story is convenient for culture but unhelpful for real human bodies. Pleasure is not an inborn script that unfolds the same way for everyone; it is a learnable, adjustable, context-sensitive skill that improves when you pay attention, slows down when you are distracted or ashamed, and changes as your body, relationships, and health change.

To learn pleasure you first have to learn to notice. Bodies send a constant flow of sensory information about pressure, stretch, temperature, rhythm, location, smell, sound, emotional tone, and people often miss it because their attention is still in work mode or in caretaker mode or in self-evaluating mode. When the mind is busy thinking, "Is this taking too long," or, "Do I look ok," or, "Is my partner getting bored," it cannot at the same time stay in contact with the small rising wave of arousal that begins in the skin. The skill, then, is to move attention from monitoring to experiencing. That shift is simple, not easy: you slow the touch, you breathe, you describe to yourself what you feel, and you let sensation become clearer.

Every piece of sexual touch is made of variables. There is the obvious variable of where you are being touched, but also how firmly, in what direction, at what speed, for how long, with which texture, and in what emotional climate. A circular, steady movement with the whole hand can feel deeply regulating to someone who came into the encounter with a tense nervous system, while the same movement, done quickly and without checking in, can feel irritating to someone who is still far from arousal. A teasing, light touch can feel delicious in the middle of high excitement, and almost meaningless at the very beginning. A kiss that lingers and includes breath can tell the body, "Stay here," in a way that five quick kisses cannot. None of this means you are difficult. It only means your erotic nervous system is precise.

Sequence matters as much as technique. Many bodies prefer to arrive at genital touch gradually, through face, scalp, neck, shoulders, chest, back, thighs, and emotional contact. That progression is not foreplay in the sense of something secondary. It is the phase during which the brain moves from neutral into erotic attention. People who were taught to hurry often skip it, land directly on genitals, and then believe that their body is "slow." In reality their body never had a chance to arrive. When the runway is longer, the takeoff is easier.

Orgasm shows up in almost every conversation about pleasure, so it helps to make it ordinary. Orgasm is a powerful and often satisfying peak, but it is not the only evidence of good sex. Some people reach orgasm easily and still feel disconnected because there was no attunement. Others do not reach orgasm at all in a given encounter but come away full, rested, and loved because the experience was generous and present. Still others orgasm more reliably alone than with a partner, which is completely consistent with what we know about arousal, because solo sex contains fewer inhibition cues. Partnered sex introduces the presence of another mind, and that mind can either support or interrupt the experience.

Research on arousal nonconcordance explains why this happens. Genital responses and subjective arousal are cousins, not twins. A vulva can lubricate in response to erotic material without the person wanting sex. A penis can become erect in the middle of a situation that is stressful or boring. The body is saying, "This is sexually relevant," while the person may be saying, "I do not want this." Both messages are valid. Desire and consent live in the mind. This is important for pleasure because it frees people from the idea that the body must always mirror the experience. You can have responsive bodies and still choose no. You can have slower bodies and still choose yes.

Solo exploration is one of the safest and most honest ways to collect data about pleasure. Many adults still feel a trace of childhood guilt about masturbation, especially if they received religious or family messages that framed it as selfish or "lesser," yet from a sexual health perspective it is a laboratory where you can test pressure, rhythm, toys, lube, fantasy, and pacing without having to manage another person's feelings. You can stop the moment something is uncomfortable. You can repeat what works. You can notice whether you prefer indirect clitoral stimulation or very focused stimulation, whether the testicles or the perineum want more touch, whether your pelvic floor tightens when you get close to orgasm, whether breathing slowly makes orgasm easier. Everything you learn there is transferable to partnered sex.

Partners, of course, cannot guess all of that. They need language, and not elegant, mysterious language, but concrete, mundane, specific language. "Stay there." "Softer." "Slower." "Do not change the rhythm when I get louder." "Use the flat of your tongue." "A little higher." "Less teeth." "Kiss my chest again first." Many people avoid that level of direction because they were taught that if sex is real it should happen without words. That is not how bodies work. Clear feedback calms performance anxiety, and once anxiety is low, both partners can enjoy the sensations instead of wondering whether they are doing it right.

Meaning is part of pleasure, sometimes the biggest part. A touch can be physically good and still fall flat if the situation feels unfair, or if you do not feel desired, or if you are still hurt about something that happened earlier. The very same touch, in the context of repair, appreciation, or celebration, can feel electric. Bodies register whether sex is motivated by duty, by fear of losing the relationship, by curiosity, or by genuine wanting. Sex that says, "I am doing this so you will not be mad," tends to be less pleasurable than sex that says, "I like you and I like what happens between us." The actions can be identical. The emotional frame changes the experience.

Fantasy sits right here, not as an escape from your partner but as a tool for feeding the accelerator. Imagination can supply novelty when the relationship is stable, can supply safety when the relationship is still building trust, can supply intensity when real life is slow, or can supply tenderness when you are tired of pressure. As long as your fantasies feel aligned with your values, they can be integrated into your erotic life. If they do not feel aligned, you can still notice which elements are arousing (is it power, is it being chosen, is it being watched, is it the setting, is it the slowness) and then build partner-friendly versions of those elements.

Pain has to be named clearly because painful sex trains the body away from pleasure. People sometimes endure penetration that hurts because they want to please a partner or because they think this is how "real" sex is supposed to be. Over time the inhibition system learns, "Sex equals pain," and it begins to lower desire in advance. This is not low libido. This is a body protecting itself. Many causes of pain can be improved: more time before penetration so that blood flow and lubrication increase, generous use of lube, different positions that take pressure off the pelvic floor, treatment for infections or endometriosis, pelvic floor physical therapy, slower movement, better communication. Once pain recedes, pleasure almost always becomes easier.

Bodies will not stay the same. Hormonal contraception, antidepressants, pregnancy, postpartum, perimenopause, menopause, chronic illness, disability, surgery, and gender-affirming treatments can all alter arousal speed, lubrication, erection, and orgasmic intensity. Those changes are not signs that you are "past it." They are signals to update technique, pacing, fantasy, and context. People who see sex as a fixed performance tend to panic when something shifts. People who see sex as an ongoing conversation tend to adapt.

The culture around us often wants to put genital intercourse at the top of the hierarchy, then oral sex, then manual sex, then cuddling, as if the value of erotic contact could be measured by how close it comes to penetration. That ranking does not match actual pleasure data. Many vulva owners orgasm more reliably from external stimulation than from penetration. Many penis owners enjoy a wide range of touch that has nothing to do with thrusting. Many couples find that long, clothed, sensual sessions produce more connection than rushed intercourse. Once you define sex as any consensual erotic activity that creates pleasure for at least one person and ideally for both, the menu expands and pressure drops.

What matters in the end is convergence: your body, in this season of life, with this partner or partners, in this context, with these beliefs, can learn to generate and receive pleasure. You do not need to match porn. You do not need to match your friends' stories. You do not need to match what you enjoyed ten years ago. You need to feel, to ask, to guide, to adjust. In the next chapter, knowing the actual anatomy of arousal will make that guidance even clearer, because you will be able to connect what you feel to the structures being stimulated and to the blood flow and nerve pathways that make orgasm possible.

Chapter 5
Anatomy for Everyone

Maps matter. When you know the geography of your own body, decisions about touch, pacing, and pleasure become easier, because you are no longer guessing in the dark. This chapter offers a tour that is practical rather than technical, accurate without being overloaded, and inclusive of the many bodies that people live in. You will see structures that most school lessons ignored, understand how arousal moves through tissues and nerves, and learn why small shifts in angle or pressure can change the entire experience.

Begin at the surface with words that name what we see. The vulva refers to the external structures, not to the internal canal. That means the labia majora and labia minora, the clitoral hood and glans, the urethral opening, the vestibule that surrounds it, and the entrance to the vagina. Colors vary widely, from pink to brown to purple, and all of that is normal. Labia can be symmetrical or not, long or short, smooth or ridged. Many discomforts people feel about appearance come from exposure to edited images rather than from medical concerns. Function does not require symmetry.

The clitoris deserves early attention because it contains the densest concentration of sensory nerve endings in the human body and, during arousal, it becomes the main generator of erotic sensation for most vulva owners. What many people call the clitoris is only the visible glans at the top of the vulva, tucked under a protective hood. The full clitoral structure extends internally in a wishbone shape, with two crura that reach along the pubic bones and two bulb-like masses of erectile tissue that flank the vaginal entrance. During arousal, blood fills these tissues and the entire complex swells, which is one reason why indirect touch can feel better at the beginning and why pressure preferences change as excitement builds. When you hear someone talk about an orgasm from the anterior vaginal wall, they are likely describing stimulation that is recruiting the internal clitoral complex through shared tissues and nerves.

Moving inward, the vagina is a muscular canal that runs from the vulvar vestibule to the cervix. At rest it measures only a few inches and sits angled toward the lower back, which means that changes in position can alter how penetration feels. The walls are normally folded, a feature called rugae, and they expand with arousal as blood flow increases and the tissue becomes more elastic. Lubrication primarily arrives through transudation, a process in which plasma seeps through the vaginal walls when they are engorged with blood. Glands near the entrance, especially the Bartholin's glands, add a small amount of slippery fluid. If lubrication varies from day to day, that reflects hormonal shifts, hydration, arousal time, and stress. Supplemental lubricant remains a valid and often very helpful tool at any age, including in young people with high desire who simply prefer more glide.

Above the vagina sits the cervix, which is the lower end of the uterus. Some people enjoy gentle contact with the cervix at high arousal, while many find direct pressure uncomfortable. Pain during deep penetration can come from the cervix being bumped repeatedly, from pelvic floor tension, from endometriosis, or from infections. None of these sensations are a test of toughness. If deep thrusting hurts, slow the rhythm, change positions to shorten the angle, or switch to external stimulation, then seek medical care when pain persists.

Ejaculatory fluid associated with vulvas often generates confusion. A set of small glands near the urethra, sometimes called Skene's or paraurethral glands, can produce fluid that exits through or near the urethral opening, and the volume can range from a trace to a gush. For some, this feels pleasurable and shows up with certain types of pressure on the anterior vaginal wall. For others, it never appears and nothing is missing. Bodies differ, and pleasure can exist with or without this response.

The pelvic floor deserves the same level of practical attention as genitals because it influences both sensation and comfort. This group of muscles forms a supportive hammock that holds the pelvic organs and helps with continence, stability, and sexual function. During arousal these muscles should be able to relax and then contract rhythmically at orgasm. When they are chronically tight, penetration can feel sharp or burning, and orgasm may be difficult to reach. When they are weak, sensations can feel dull and leaks can occur during exertion. Pelvic floor physical therapy is a valuable option for all genders, and can improve pain, sensitivity, and function at every age.

Shift now to the external genital anatomy for penis owners. The penis includes the shaft, the glans at the tip, and in many bodies a foreskin that protects the glans. Under the skin live three columns of erectile tissue. Two corpora cavernosa run along the top and help create firmness, and one corpus spongiosum surrounds the urethra and expands into the glans. During arousal, increased blood flow fills these tissues while outflow is restricted, leading to erection. Sensation concentrates on the frenulum, the ridge where the foreskin attaches, and on the glans. Circumcision changes the distribution of sensitivity by removing the foreskin and exposing the glans, which then develops a different skin texture over time. Pleasure remains available with or without foreskin, although touch preferences may differ.

Testes and scrotum contribute to sexual experience through both hormonal production and sensation. The testicles produce testosterone and sperm, and the scrotum contains smooth muscle that contracts and relaxes to regulate temperature. For many, gentle handling of the scrotum, perineum, and the cords above the testes adds intensity. The perineum, the area between genitals and anus, overlies deep structures and nerves, which is why firm pressure there can feel unexpectedly arousing.

Internally, two organs often enter conversations about pleasure: the prostate and the urethra. The prostate surrounds the urethra just below the bladder and contributes fluid to semen. Stimulation through the rectum or through rhythmic pressure on the perineum can create intense sensations for some penis owners. Others feel nothing special. Hygiene, consent, slow pacing, and lubrication are nonnegotiable when exploring anal touch, and no one is required to enjoy it for their sexuality to be complete.

A brief look at arousal physiology connects these structures. Sexual excitement begins with signals from the brain, often in response to touch, fantasy, smell, sight, memory, or context. Those signals travel through autonomic nerves to increase blood flow in erectile tissues. For vulvas, that means swelling of the clitoris, vestibular bulbs, and labia, and increased lubrication within the vagina. For penises, that means firming through the corpora cavernosa and spongiosum, and increased sensitivity of the glans and frenulum. Heart rate and breathing rise, skin flushes, and muscles prepare for rhythmic contractions. After peak intensity, arousal gradually resolves as blood flow returns to baseline.

Nerve pathways explain why people reach orgasm through different routes. The pudendal nerve provides much of the sensation for external genitals in all bodies. The pelvic and hypo-gastric nerves carry signals from deeper structures, including the cervix, uterus, and prostate. There is also evidence that the vagus nerve can transmit pelvic sensation, which helps explain orgasm in people with certain spinal injuries. When someone reports orgasms from clitoral touch, penile shaft stimulation, anal play, or deep pressure against the anterior vaginal wall, they are using overlapping networks rather than separate "types" of orgasm. The variation is one reason people benefit from changing position, angle, or rhythm to find the path that best recruits their available nerves.

Language about the so-called G-spot has led to confusion for decades. Rather than hunting for a single button, think of a re-gion on the anterior vaginal wall that shares tissues and nerves with the deeper clitoral network and the urethral complex. Some people feel strong pleasure from firm, rhythmic pressure in that region, especially when well aroused and well lubri-cated, and others feel nothing notable. Both experiences fit normal anatomy. What matters is not the label but whether the sensation feels good for the person whose body it is.

Trans bodies and bodies undergoing hormonal or surgical care belong fully in this anatomy. Estrogen, testosterone, and puberty blockers change skin thickness, hair growth, lubrica-tion, erectile responsiveness, and distribution of body fat. Gen-der-affirming surgeries, such as vaginoplasty, phalloplasty, metoidioplasty, chest reconstruction, or breast augmentation, create new relationships between nerves and tissues. Sensation can be present, absent, or altered, and it often evolves over time as healing continues and as the brain remaps touch. Pleasure remains possible in every configuration, although discovery may take patience and deliberate exploration.

Hormonal transitions outside of gender-affirming care also reshape sexual tissues. During perimenopause and menopause, lower estrogen can reduce elasticity and natural lubrication, which can lead to irritation if penetration is rushed. Local estrogen therapies, generous external stimulation, and lubricant use can restore comfort and sensation. During pregnancy and postpartum, increased blood flow and shifts in pelvic floor tone can change sensitivity. Antidepressants and other medications can influence arousal and orgasm by altering neurotransmitters. None of these changes erase sexuality. They do invite updates to technique, pace, and context.

Positioning deserves a practical paragraph because anatomy is three-dimensional and angle matters. Many people find that small adjustments, such as placing a pillow under hips, changing the tilt of the pelvis, or rotating the body slightly, transform deep pressure from uncomfortable to satisfying. In penetrative sex with a penis or toy, positions that allow the receiver to control depth and tempo often improve comfort by protecting tender areas. In oral sex, head and neck support can make longer sessions pleasurable rather than tiring. These are anatomical choices rather than preferences that carry meaning about who is dominant or submissive, and they often matter more than anyone expects.

Touch techniques also benefit from anatomical thinking. Clitoral glans stimulation can be exquisitely intense for some and overwhelming for others, especially at the beginning. In those cases, indirect touch to the hood or to the labia minora provides sensation while the tissues warm up. On penises, steady strokes that include the frenulum often work well early, while varied grip and rhythm maintain interest as arousal climbs. Across bodies, a consistent tempo tends to be more effective than constant novelty once someone is close to orgasm, because nerve firing patterns respond to repetition.

Anatomy includes smell, taste, and natural fluids, which carry strong cultural messages. Healthy genitals have a scent. Semen varies in volume and thickness, urethral pre-ejaculate can appear before orgasm, and vaginal lubrication changes through the cycle. Clean bodies that have been allowed to be bodies are not dirty. If a scent feels distracting, address context with showers together, different timing, or breathable fabrics. Shame shrinks pleasure more than any normal smell ever could.

Strength and flexibility through the hips, lower back, and thighs influence sexual comfort, which is still an anatomical issue rather than a fitness ideal. Simple movements that lengthen hip flexors, mobilize the lower spine, and relax the inner thighs can expand the range of positions that feel good. Relaxation practices that lower overall muscle tension make genital blood flow more efficient and reduce pain. Think of this as tuning the instrument you already have.

No tour would be complete without a reminder about variation. All bodies deviate from textbook diagrams. Some clitoral hoods are tight and benefit from gentle retraction during arousal, while others retract easily. Some vaginal canals are angled more sharply toward the back, which makes certain positions feel better. Some penises curve upward, downward, or to one side, which changes how pressure lands and can create special pleasure with the right alignment. None of this requires correction unless there is pain or functional limitation. Variation creates opportunities for custom pleasure.

The point of learning anatomy is not to memorize Latin names. The point is to gain enough clarity that you can steer. When you know that the clitoral network is large, you stop trying to force pleasure through penetration that is not producing sensation. When you understand that the cervix sits shallow in some positions, you make adjustments rather than deciding your body is broken. When you remember that nerves bring sensation from multiple routes, you stop ranking orgasms and start collecting them. Knowledge does not kill mystery. It frees you to spend less time guessing and more time enjoying.

In the next chapter we will step away from tissues and look at the brain again, focusing on emotion, attachment, and memory, because anatomy describes what touch can do, while the mind determines how that touch is translated into meaning. Together they form the terrain where sexual wellbeing grows.

Chapter 6
The Brain on Sex: Emotion, Attachment, and Memory

Desire begins in a body, yet it is organized by a brain that never stops evaluating context, meaning, and risk. When people say that sex is in the head, they are not dismissing the body. They are acknowledging that every sensation passes through attention, emotion, and memory before it becomes pleasure. If you have ever felt aroused in a scene that made narrative sense to you and completely flat in a scene that looked erotic on paper, you have witnessed how the brain sets the terms for the body.

Arousal involves several neural systems working at once. Attention has to narrow toward the erotic target rather than staying scattered among chores, worries, and notifications. Motivation has to rise enough to move your body toward touch. Reward circuits have to predict that the outcome will feel good. In parallel, inhibition systems keep scanning for danger or cost. Neurochemistry coordinates this dance. Dopamine increases when something seems exciting or promising. Norepinephrine heightens alertness and can focus attention on the erotic object. Oxytocin increases feelings of bonding and lowers the sense of social threat when there is trust. Endogenous opioids create a sense of satisfaction and soothe pain. Serotonin modulates mood and can either support or dampen desire depending on balance and timing. Cortisol rises with stress and can push the system back toward vigilance. None of these chemicals operate as on-off switches. They interact with history and with what the situation means to you.

Attachment patterns shape those meanings before you ever arrive at a bedroom. If early relationships taught you that closeness is safe and that separation is tolerable because people return, your nervous system tends to settle more quickly in intimate scenes. Many adults call this secure attachment. If early relationships were inconsistent and you learned to track other people closely in order to stay connected, your nervous system may enter sex with a watchful quality and use sex to seek reassurance. Many adults call this an anxious pattern. If early relationships taught you that closeness is risky and that you should rely on yourself because others are intrusive or unreliable, your nervous system may prefer distance and may use sex without deep emotional access. Many adults call this an avoidant pattern. These are not diagnoses and they are not fixed destinies. They are tendencies that show up in how quickly or slowly your body relaxes enough to feel pleasure with another person.

Emotion sets the tone for arousal because the brain tags experiences with feeling before you fully interpret them. A raised voice from a partner can shift your system into mild defense even if you tell yourself not to be sensitive. A kind message in the middle of a hard day can make your chest loosen in ways that later translate into receptivity. This is the groundwork for what sex therapists call co-regulation. Two nervous systems in a room influence each other. When one person slows breathing, softens voice, and approaches with curiosity, the other person's physiology often follows. When one person carries agitation and moves quickly, the other person's system may brace or check out. Many couples discover that foreplay begins long before touch and that tone, timing, and small gestures are neurobiological interventions rather than romantic extras.

Memory links all of this together. The brain is a prediction machine. It uses past experience to forecast how the next moment will feel. If you had several erotic encounters that ended with pressure, criticism, or pain, your brain will predict more of the same and will preemptively lower arousal. If you had a sequence of experiences where you felt chosen, respected, and satisfied, your brain will predict pleasure and will begin preparing the body as soon as cues appear. This is why a single disappointing night can feel larger than it should. The mind does not simply store events; it builds expectations.

The good news in memory science is reconsolidation. When you recall an old learning in a safe context and then experience a different outcome, the brain can update the meaning attached to that learning. A person who learned that asking for slower touch leads to mockery can, in a new relationship, ask for slower touch and receive care instead, and the brain will gradually retag that action as safe. A person who learned that their arousal is too slow and therefore shameful can, with a patient partner, go at their own pace and feel wanted anyway, and the brain will soften the old conclusion. You do not erase the original memory. You add a stronger, updated version that becomes easier to access.

Performance anxiety shows up here as an interference in prediction. When the mind begins monitoring arousal rather than experiencing it, it recruits cognitive resources that could otherwise process sensation and pleasure. A penis owner who becomes preoccupied with erection pulls attention away from touch and toward evaluation, which increases sympathetic arousal in a way that conflicts with erection. A vulva owner who becomes preoccupied with lubrication or with whether orgasm will happen pulls attention away from sensation and toward judgment, which increases muscle tension in a way that conflicts with orgasm. The antidote is not to stop thinking by force. The antidote is to redirect attention to specific sensory channels and to use breath as a metronome for presence, because breath gives the mind a neutral task while the body catches up.

Fantasy enters as a tool for attention. Erotic imagery has the power to supply the brain with context, story, and anticipation that might be missing in the moment. Many people use fantasy to bridge from neutral into aroused states, not because their partner is lacking, but because the brain sometimes needs narrative fuel to engage the reward system. If a fantasy conflicts with your values, you can still notice which ingredients are arousing, such as being sought after, being in control, being cared for, or being in a novel setting, and then build partner-friendly versions that carry those same ingredients without the parts that trouble you.

The nervous system states known as sympathetic and parasympathetic set boundaries for erotic function. Sympathetic activation helps with excitement and focus at moderate levels, yet too much sympathetic activation tips into fight or flight and squeezes out pleasure. Parasympathetic tone supports relaxation, genital blood flow, and orgasmic release when it is strong enough. People often talk about wanting more desire while living in conditions that keep the sympathetic system high all day. Practices that increase parasympathetic tone, such as slow exhale breathing, warm baths, unhurried kissing, laughter, and gentle eye contact, are not clichés. They are ways to move physiology into a zone where arousal can actually rise.

Attachment shows up again in how people repair after sexual misses. A securely oriented person tends to interpret a partner's low interest as about context. An anxiously oriented person often interprets the same event as a sign of impending loss. An avoidantly oriented person may withdraw faster and may dislike conversation about the miss. The repair matters because it prevents the memory system from filing the event under danger. When couples name what went wrong without blame and plan the next attempt with different conditions, the brain stores the night as a solvable problem rather than as a threat.

Novelty deserves careful treatment because reward circuits respond strongly to new stimuli, yet attachment thrives on familiarity. Many long-term couples struggle with this dynamic. They want stability and they want excitement. The brain can support both when novelty is contextual rather than interpersonal. A new setting, a new time of day, a new sequence, a new script negotiated through fantasy, or a new agreement about who initiates can increase dopamine without threatening the bond. People often assume that novelty means adding people or adding risk. Neurobiology says that novelty means changing prediction just enough that attention wakes up.

Trauma alters many of these pathways by teaching the inhibition system to be vigilant. Intrusive memories, startle responses, numbness, pelvic floor tension, and dissociation are not stubborn personality traits. They are protective strategies that became automated. Healing begins with safety and choice, then adds gradual exposure to sensation in ways that stay within tolerance. Some survivors prefer to reclaim erotic touch directly. Others prefer sensual, non-genital explorations for a long time. The brain will not be bullied into pleasure. It will return when conditions are right and when the person is allowed to set the pace.

Medications and medical conditions affect the brain's sexual circuits in ways that tend to be reversible with adjustment. Antidepressants can lower libido or delay orgasm by altering serotonin. Some blood pressure medicines influence erection by changing vascular tone. Pain conditions consume attention and bias prediction toward discomfort. None of these factors mean that desire is over. They mean that you will need collaboration between medical care, behavioral strategies, and patient partners so that prediction can move from cost to reward again.

Aftercare may look unromantic on paper and feels essential in practice because it cements memories of safety and connection. A few minutes of quiet holding, water, a snack, or a short conversation that says, "This worked, this part could be different next time," gives the brain closure. Closure helps the system mark the encounter as complete and positive, which increases the chance that desire will rise again later. Without aftercare, especially in intense scenes, the nervous system may remain activated and interpret the arousal peak as stress rather than as pleasure.

When people understand that sex is not a single reflex but a coordinated interaction among attention, emotion, attachment, prediction, and inhibition, they stop blaming themselves for responses that make sense. You are not failing if your mind needs reassurance for your body to respond. You are not failing if a hard week pulls your attention away from sex. You are not failing if your system prefers to warm up through fantasy or through slow eye contact and touch. The brain is doing what it is designed to do. Your job is to give it reasons to predict that erotic experiences are safe, meaningful, and rewarding, so that it will help your body move toward them.

Chapter 7
Shame, Myths, and Sexual Scripts

Every culture distributes stories about sex that feel like facts. Those stories become scripts that run quietly in the background until someone stops to examine them, and by the time adults arrive in intimate relationships, the script often feels like a rulebook. If your mind has ever supplied lines such as real sex means penetration, good women do not initiate, real men never decline, or loving couples climax together, you have heard the script at work. Health improves when scripts are treated as drafts that can be revised to fit real bodies, real values, and real relationships.

Shame grows from the same soil as those scripts and settles not only on actions but on identity. A person who internalized purity rules may still believe that pleasure reduces worth. A person who learned that sexual conquest proves value may feel defective when desire dips. Queer and trans people who spent years shielding erotic life to stay safe may find secrecy lingering even in supportive contexts. Shame does not merely say that something you did was wrong. It says that who you are is unacceptable, and once that message attaches to sexuality, the body often lowers arousal because exposure feels dangerous.

Myths reinforce shame by pretending that variability does not exist. The myth of virginity as a clear, measurable condition remains common, despite the fact that anatomy offers no reliable sign and lived experience is more complex than a before-and-after line. The myth that penetration sits at the top of a hierarchy of acts keeps many couples stuck in routines that do not match their bodies, even when external stimulation would bring more pleasure. The myth that men are always ready and women are always slower erases same-gender couples and pushes people into roles that do not reflect how their systems actually work. The myth that porn depicts typical sex confuses a performance edited for effect with education, which invites comparison instead of curiosity.

Scripts can either support or punish. A supportive script says that sex is a place for consent, mutual care and honesty, exploration, and pleasure that adapts to context. A punitive script says that sex is a test you pass or fail, that frequency proves love, that orgasm is a score, that bodies must match a narrow template, and that speaking up ruins the mood. People rarely choose punitive scripts on purpose. They absorb them from families, faith communities, media, and peers, and once absorbed, the script polices from inside your own head.

The work of unscripting begins with clear language. Sit down alone or with a partner and write out the rules you were taught: what counts as "real sex," who should initiate, how often a couple should have sex, what bodies should look like, whose pleasure matters most, what kinds of touch are permitted, what topics must never be spoken. Then ask fuller, parallel questions that invite reflection. What do I currently believe counts as sex, and why did I learn that? Who do I expect to initiate, and where did that expectation come from? How often do I think a couple should have sex, and does that frequency match our lives right now? What do I believe about how bodies should look, and who gave me that belief? Whose pleasure do I treat as central, and does that fit my values? Which forms of touch do I consider off limits, and is the origin of that rule ethical or simply inherited? When you examine the answers, many rules lose their force in the light of day. Others may carry values you want to keep, such as fidelity, mutual care and honesty, or privacy, but they need to be translated into language that fits your current relationship rather than the household where you learned them.

Body scripts are powerful because images repeat them every day. When bodies deviate from the narrow template of youth, thinness, and high stamina, people start hiding angles, keeping lights off, refusing oral sex, or rushing encounters to get them over with. Performance replaces sensation, and an imagined audience replaces a present partner. The corrective is not instant self-love. The corrective is treating your actual body as eligible for pleasure today and building experiences where being seen leads to kindness, which teaches the nervous system that exposure is safe.

Gender scripts still shape behavior even in couples that consider themselves egalitarian. Men taught to lead, provide, and penetrate can feel trapped when they need slowness, comfort, or help with initiation. Women taught to accommodate, please, and receive can feel erased when they want to chase, to direct, or to prefer external stimulation. Nonbinary and trans partners are often edited out of inherited scripts entirely, which is its own form of erasure. Couples who thrive tend to compose a shared script that lets each person be a full human rather than a role. That script clarifies who initiates and when, which words affirm, which kinds of touch feel good, which activities are off the table for now, and how each partner will say no.

Porn deserves careful context. For some, it functions as arousal fuel and a space for private exploration. For others, it becomes a syllabus that trains expectations for bodies, timing, endurance, and consent in ways that do not map onto real intimacy. The issue is not arousal in response to visual material; human attention often responds to novelty. The issue is mistaking edited performance for instruction. People who integrate porn without harm usually frame it as fiction, discuss it openly when partnered, avoid material that conflicts with their ethics, and make sure that real-life sexual education comes from research, conversation, and feedback between partners.

Because shame thrives in secrecy, wise disclosure can be corrective. You can tell a partner that you were taught to avoid sex and that you are learning to claim pleasure. You can say that you were taught to serve and that you want reciprocity. You can admit that you were taught never to decline and that you sometimes need to. The goal is not confession for drama. The goal is to let someone see the script you carry so that they stop taking your responses personally and begin collaborating in a rewrite. Collaboration produces experiences that contradict the old narrative. Contradictory experiences become the new evidence your mind uses to predict safety.

Religious and moral commitments belong in the conversation with respect. Many people hold values about sex that matter deeply, and those values can coexist with pleasure when they are framed around care and consent rather than control. A person can hold a belief that sex belongs in committed relationships and still prioritize mutual delight. A person can value modesty and still communicate exquisite detail about what feels good. A person can choose monogamy and still cultivate novelty through creativity rather than new partners. Ethics organized around dignity, agency, and responsibility tend to support erotic life rather than restrict it.

Language shapes expectation. When couples shift from outcome language to process language, pressure drops and curiosity increases. Instead of asking whether they finished, they ask whether they felt close, whether they listened, whether they explored. Instead of saying that one partner never wants sex, they say that one accelerator needs more warm up and the other brake is sensitive to stress, so together they design conditions that work for both. Instead of calling everything before penetration "foreplay," they call it warm up or connection, which tells the brain that these activities are part of sex rather than delays.

Repairing shame benefits from private practices that build self-compassion and from social spaces that normalize honest talk. Some people write responses to the inner script in a steadier voice. Others pair mirror time with gentle touch to connect sight and acceptance. Still others choose therapy that treats sexual concerns as health concerns. Friends who speak plainly about sex without bragging or shaming create a healthier ambient script. Parents who name bodies accurately and answer questions without panic give children a foundation for consent and agency. Healthcare providers who ask about comfort and function signal that sexual health deserves clinical attention. Media that includes diverse bodies and diverse pleasures expands expectations. Each of these inputs helps replace punitive rules with humane ones.

Practice makes new scripts real. Couples who decide to move away from a penetration-centered model might plan evenings focused on external touch, oral sex, mutual masturbation, or sensual massage, not as consolation prizes but as legitimate expressions of intimacy. Individuals who want to remove shame about fantasy might share broad themes and discover relief rather than threat. Partners who wish to rebuild initiation might agree on windows of time, signals, and types of approach that reduce pressure. Repetition creates data, data builds confidence, and confidence quiets shame.

When myths and scripts lose their grip, sex stops feeling like a test and starts feeling like a place to exercise agency and play. Health here does not require meeting an idealized scene. It requires alignment between values and behavior, between what a body can offer today and what is asked of it, between how you want to treat others and how you ask to be treated. That alignment is the opposite of shame. It is permission. It is the context where desire can grow.

Chapter 8
Communication That Actually Works

People often say they are bad at talking about sex, yet they speak about it all the time without noticing. They sigh when a hand moves too fast. They turn slightly away when an approach feels abrupt. They go quiet after a night that missed the mark. Bodies hold long conversations that partners never translate. The project of sexual communication is to bring those messages into words that are clear, kind, and specific, so that touch can follow accurate instructions rather than guesses.

Begin with a principle that changes the room before any sentence is spoken. Conversation goes better when the goal is collaboration instead of proof. If you walk in trying to prove that you are right or that your partner is wrong, the body gears up to defend. If you walk in trying to design a better experience for both of you, the body relaxes into problem solving. Relaxed bodies listen. Tense bodies litigate. The difference shows up in tone, in posture, in how quickly people interrupt, and in whether anyone can remember what was said.

Setting is part of the message. Couples frequently attempt high stakes sexual talks at the end of the day, in bed, under covers, with fatigue already humming in the background. Those talks often collapse into frustration or silence. Mornings on weekends work better for many pairs. A walk after dinner works for others. A parked car can work when there are roommates or children at home. What matters is that both of you feel unhurried and clothed, because nudity during difficult topics can activate shame or pressure. Choose a neutral place, agree on a time boundary, and tell each other what success would look like for this one conversation. Success might be learning one new preference, or agreeing on a plan for the next week, or repairing a small rupture from last night.

Language does most of the heavy lifting once you have a place and a time. The sentence that reaches a partner's body contains three elements. It names a concrete observation. It describes impact in first person. It makes a specific request that can happen soon. Compare two versions. You never touch me unless you want sex, which lands as a judgment and invites rebuttal, and When you only touch me during sex, I feel distant during the day, and I would love a long kiss when you get home, before we talk about anything practical. The second version gives a map and a time. Bodies like maps.

Specificity signals respect. A partner cannot follow the instruction be more romantic. They can follow, text me once during the day to say you are thinking of me, then kiss me in the kitchen before logistics. A partner cannot follow, initiate more. They can follow, look me in the eyes and say I want you, then wait for me to answer before you touch my chest. When you ask for what you want in this level of detail, you are not micro-managing. You are translating your nervous system into plain English.

Feedback during sex is its own language. Many adults avoid it because they fear sounding clinical or critical. The irony is that bodies become more erotic when the mind knows it is on the right track. You can practice small phrases that keep sensation flowing while steering touch: softer, slower, stay there, a little higher, keep the same rhythm, use your whole hand, less pressure, kiss my neck again, pause for a second and breathe with me. Partners who learn to offer and receive such guidance tend to report fewer misses and more ease. The guiding partner feels empowered rather than performed upon. The receiving partner enjoys certainty rather than guessing.

Listening creates arousal in ways people underestimate. Not the passive kind where you wait for your turn to speak, but the kind where you mirror what you heard and check that you got it. I am hearing that late at night is the hardest time for you, and you want more warm up earlier in the evening. Did I get that right. The other person's shoulders often drop in that moment. Your accuracy removes the need to argue for reality. Once reality is shared, solutions appear.

Timing of difficult feedback matters as much as wording. Directing touch in the moment keeps a scene alive. Debriefing technique at midnight can flood a partner with shame. You can postpone elaboration to the next day and frame it as design, not critique. Yesterday, when you changed rhythm right before I was close, I lost the wave. Next time, if I am louder or breathing faster, that means keep everything the same for a bit. That sentence does not accuse. It instructs a future.

Initiation is a recurring pain point in long bonds, and it deserves as much craft as technique. Couples who wait for spontaneous desire to line up perfectly tend to wait a long time. You can make initiation a shared project by agreeing on windows that fit your bodies. Some pairs choose early evening twice a week. Others choose Saturday morning and one floating time. Inside those windows, the higher-desire partner can lead without fear of rejection, and the responsive-desire partner can agree to begin without promising a specific outcome. Beginning might mean a shower together, or a nap that turns into touch, or a massage that may or may not become sex. The promise is presence and curiosity, not a performance. Presence invites desire. Pressure scares it away.

Because desire ebbs and flows, the word no needs a companion so that it does not close the door. No, tonight I am not up for penetration, and I would love a long make-out on the couch. No, my head hurts, and I can hold you while you touch yourself and kiss you when you finish. No, not now, and yes to tomorrow morning after coffee. These are honest ways to protect a boundary while protecting the connection. Partners who learn to offer a path instead of a wall discover that refusal stops feeling like rejection and starts feeling like care.

Consent lives at the center of communication and must be practical, not theoretical. Practical consent is built on signals that are easy to say in the middle of arousal. A pair can agree on green for keep going, yellow for slow down, red for stop and reset. They can agree that red is followed by water and holding, not questions and defense. They can agree on periodic check-ins that sound like Is this still good or Do you want more of this. These simple scripts keep both partners in the same scene and teach nervous systems that boundaries will be respected.

Repair is the skill that keeps conversations from becoming rare events you dread. Misses will happen even in loving relationships. Someone will move too fast. Someone will go quiet and then resent it. Someone will say yes from obligation and feel sad afterward. The next day is an opportunity to prevent the memory from turning into a rule. I pushed last night, and I am sorry. I want to slow down next time and let you set the pace. Are you open to trying again on Saturday afternoon. This kind of repair maintains trust. Trust keeps arousal possible.

Many couples benefit from a weekly check-in that includes sex along with logistics. Ten minutes on Sundays can change a month. You review the previous week for one thing that went well and one thing to adjust. You schedule the next low-stress window for intimacy. You confirm any medical or parenting constraints. You ask a small question such as What would make you feel more wanted this week or What would make starting easier. The point is not bureaucracy. The point is to keep erotic life on the agenda so that it does not have to shout to be noticed.

Text can be a powerful channel when used with intention. A brief message midweek can prime attention without creating pressure. I keep thinking about your laugh last night. I want to kiss you when you get home. I am free Saturday after lunch and want to be close. These sentences supply a story that the brain can hold during the day. When bodies meet later, they are not starting from zero. People who worry that planning will kill spontaneity usually discover the opposite. Planning removes obstacles so that spontaneity can show up.

Childhood lessons sneak into sexual talk unless you name them. Some adults learned that asking for needs is selfish. Others learned that saying no makes love disappear. Others learned that leadership equals worth and adapt poorly. Naming the old rule begins to loosen it. I learned to be low maintenance, which made me quiet. I am practicing asking and I will feel awkward at first. A partner who hears that line can support the experiment instead of misreading the awkwardness as disinterest.

Fantasy deserves careful communication because it often carries the keys to acceleration. You do not need to narrate every image. You can offer themes that your partner can act on. I get aroused when you choose me with words. I get aroused when you slow me down and hold my face. I get aroused when you ask permission and then take charge inside my yes. I get aroused when I am given a task and praised for doing it. Themes convert to actions. Actions convert to sensation. Once a theme is known, couples can build scenes that fit values and still feel vivid.

Conversations about porn and toys are easier when framed as design choices that protect the relationship. You can ask what role porn plays for each of you and whether there are categories that work or do not work. You can decide on times when porn use is off the table because you want to reserve attention for each other. You can agree on a plan for introducing a vibrator, a sleeve, or a plug, and try it together before using it alone, or the reverse, depending on comfort. The goal is transparency so that ordinary tools do not become secrets.

Medical topics belong inside sexual talk, not beside it. Antidepressants that delay orgasm, hormonal contraception that changes lubrication, blood pressure medication that alters erection, pelvic pain that narrows options, ADHD that makes sustained attention unpredictable, autism that changes sensory thresholds, trauma histories that set smaller windows of tolerance, all of these require language. A partner cannot adapt to needs that were never named. You can say, my medication makes orgasm slow, so I would love longer warm up and consistent rhythm. You can say, pelvic floor therapy is part of our plan because I want penetration to feel safe again. You can say, eye contact is hard for me when sensation is intense, so please do not take it personally if I look away.

Neurodivergent couples do well with more explicit agreements about signal, sequence, and sensory load. A written script can look unromantic in theory and produce better sex in practice. The script might list the order for a scene, which kinds of touch are on the menu, which phrases are welcome, when to pause for a breath, and how to end. You can still improvise. The script removes guesswork that would otherwise keep one partner in their head.

Long distance partners have their own communication art. Erotic attention can be nurtured through voice, through photo exchange that follows agreed limits, through shared fantasy written in a private document, through coordinated solo sessions that end with a debrief. The same rules apply. Be specific about what you want to hear. Name boundaries before play begins. Offer aftercare even by text so that the body receives closure.

Rejection is inevitable and needs ritual so that it does not corrode desire. The person declining can offer warmth and an alternative: I am a no tonight, and I would love a bath together and a back rub, or I am a no now, and I am a yes on Friday morning. The person receiving the no can respond with grace: Thank you for telling me, I will ask again another day, and then actually ask again without withdrawing affection. The ritual prevents no from meaning I do not want you. It begins to mean I am caring for my body and our connection.

Gratitude amplifies what works and should be spoken out loud. People often think appreciation is obvious. It is not. Say, I loved the way you kissed my shoulder before you moved lower. Say, when you asked if I wanted more pressure, I felt safe. Say, the message you sent in the afternoon changed my whole evening. Appreciation teaches your partner which actions matter and motivates more of them. The loop becomes self-sustaining.

When conflict appears, return to first principles. Name the pattern rather than the person. We fall into a loop where you initiate late and I say no, then we both feel alone. Suggest an experiment instead of a verdict. What if we try mornings twice a week for a month and see what changes. Set a review date so that neither of you feels trapped. On the first Sunday next month, let us talk about what worked. Experiments soothe the nervous system because they limit risk and promise data.

Polyamorous and open structures require even more communication, because the number of nervous systems increases. Agreements about time, disclosure, safer sex, and aftercare keep the primary bond from feeling abandoned. Check-ins after dates, clear plans for sex health testing, and invitations to name jealousy without shame create the stability that keeps erotic life alive for everyone involved. None of this removes the need to design conditions for desire inside the central relationship. New partners do not fix old brakes. Skills do.

If your relationship includes a history of hurt around sex, whether betrayal, pressure, or a long season of avoidance, you can still build conversations that support repair. Start smaller than you think you should. Begin with a scene that does not risk retraumatizing either person, such as a clothed massage with clear signals. Debrief afterward in a format that honors both sides. I felt close when you asked permission before you moved under my shirt. I felt scared when you sped up. Next time I want to say yellow sooner. These details rebuild trust faster than grand promises.

Parents often ask how to talk when privacy is rare. The answer is to plan like you would plan anything precious. Put a lock on a door. Trade childcare with friends once a month. Put on a movie for the kids and take a shower together for ten minutes. Use car dates. Send a message at lunch that sets up a small scene after bedtime. Schedule a morning off work once a quarter. These are not luxuries. They are communication choices that say our erotic life matters enough to earn calendar space.

You can keep a private record if that suits your mind. Some people keep an intimacy log with brief notes about what worked and what to try next. Others keep a list titled sentences that worked on me, which they hand to a partner as a gift. Others keep a menu of initiation options that feel good, arranged from soft to direct. None of these habits replace spontaneity. They feed it by giving both of you more ways to succeed.

When partners practice this kind of communication, sex changes even before anyone learns new techniques. Pressure drops because nobody is guessing. Safety rises because boundaries and wishes are spoken in advance. Curiosity returns because there is room for questions rather than performances. Desire likes those conditions. It tends to show up sooner and stay longer when the mind trusts the room.

The work is not glamorous on paper. You choose a good time, you use accurate words, you ask for one small thing, you listen for the body under your partner's sentences, you repair misses, you appreciate wins, you plan the next touch. That is all. That is enough. Conversation becomes foreplay because it clears a path that bodies can follow. When you make that path together, sex stops feeling like a test and starts feeling like a place where two nervous systems meet, learn, and play.

Chapter 9
Partnered Sex: Connection, Timing, and Mismatched Desire

Partnership brings another nervous system into the room, with its own accelerators and brakes, its own history of tenderness and injury, its own images of what sex should mean. That second nervous system can feel like an obstacle when rhythms do not match, yet it can also become the richest source of erotic energy you will ever know, because two bodies can share labor, shape context together, and create stories that no one could build alone. The puzzle is to design conditions that welcome both people as they are, on the real day they are living, and then to let desire grow inside that design.

Connection starts long before any clothes come off. Every small action outside the bedroom teaches the body what to expect when the bedroom door closes, so marital logistics are not merely chores. They are prelude. When someone carries the morning with grace, checks in during the day with a message that says I am thinking of you, notices the unfinished task and finishes it without being asked, or circles back to repair a sharp tone from yesterday, the mind stores a prediction: this person is on my side. That prediction travels with you into touch. People often tell me that a kiss feels different after a day spent feeling partnered, and there is physiology behind that report, because an organism that expects relief rather than demand relaxes sooner, and relaxed organisms feel more.

Timing is the next gate. Many couples slide into a late night default because the house becomes quiet only after bedtime, then wonder why sex keeps feeling like one more task. The brain by that hour has already moved toward sleep, which means attention is thinner and patience is short. Respecting physiology can change everything without forcing anyone into grand gestures. Some pairs walk after dinner and let movement loosen conversation that later turns into a shower and a slower approach. Others block one early morning each week for contact that does not have to rush. Others look for windows during weekends, when the nervous system is less crowded with work alarms. If late night is truly the only time, preparation matters. Screens go away, lights dim to cue the body toward parasympathetic tone, and there is a deliberate decompression before any sexual invitation appears, because no one transitions well from spreadsheets to sex in a single step.

Mismatched desire is the rule rather than the exception. People who believe that a healthy couple should want sex at the same time and in the same amount set themselves up for conflict. The dual control model offers a friendlier map. One partner's accelerator may ping often even during stressful weeks, while the other's accelerator may need more context. One person may carry a brake that responds strongly to mess or noise, while the other barely notices the sink. A workable story describes two valid systems that require different entry points. The person who experiences frequent spontaneous desire can learn to initiate in ways that feel like an invitation rather than a test. The person who experiences responsive desire can agree to begin scenes more often without precommitting to a particular outcome, trusting that desire often grows once there is warm up, privacy, and kindness.

Initiation style often matters more than frequency. Many relationships rely on a single approach that works for one body and not for the other, then interpret the lack of success as rejection. If your partner needs time to shift roles, beginning with conversation that has nothing to do with logistics and everything to do with noticing them can work, then let your hands move to shoulders or hair, then pause to see whether the mind is joining the body. If your partner craves directness, say what you want with eyes and words, name a plan for the next ten minutes, and leave space for a yes that is freely given. Some people are moved by playfulness. Others respond to reverence. Some respond best to being asked whether they want to be approached slowly or quickly, then having that choice honored. When initiation fits the receiver's nervous system, desire feels invited rather than demanded.

A shared menu of sex helps with both initiation and consent. Treat the phrase have sex as too vague to be useful and name specific options that count as complete encounters. A long session of external touch that includes orgasm for one or both people counts. Mutual masturbation that involves eye contact and praise counts. Oral sex without penetration counts. Penetration for a short time with generous lube and no goal for orgasm counts. An evening that begins with massage and ends with sleep because the slower partner's body stayed at warmth, not fire, still counts as intimacy. When couples expand what qualifies, they discover more ways to say yes on nights when a former all or nothing standard would have produced a no.

Touch quality keeps partnered sex from going stale, because attention adapts quickly to repetition. Variety does not require acrobatics or new costumes every week. It asks for curiosity about pressure, rhythm, angle, and sequence. A receiver who tends to tense can settle when touch is firm and steady across large areas before becoming focused. A receiver who tends to drift can reengage when rhythm changes slightly at predictable intervals. The person giving touch can watch for breath, sound, and micro-movements, then mirror them, because mirroring brings the nervous systems into sync. Many partners change something exactly when the other is close. A simple rule prevents that miss. Once you suspect that the wave is rising, keep the same pressure, location, and rhythm until the receiver asks for change or you feel release.

Power dynamics are always present. Some partners enjoy scenes that include authority and surrender within clear consent; others prefer egalitarian energy at all times. Even in couples that do not play explicitly, power sneaks in through who initiates, who sets pace, and whose preferences receive more airtime. Sex becomes labor for the person who constantly adapts while the other remains unexamined. Counterweights help. Alternate who leads for a month. Choose a season where the historically slower desiring partner sets every pace, with the understanding that the faster partner will enjoy a different kind of pleasure, one rooted in attunement rather than in frequency. Build scenes where the person who usually gives receives as a deliberate practice rather than as a rare treat. Power that is chosen can feel intensely erotic. Power that is assumed often erodes desire.

Pain and comfort are shared responsibilities. When penetration hurts, the couple has a pain problem, not a motivation problem. Pushing through does not build resilience. Pushing through trains the inhibition system to predict harm and lowers desire later. Partners who protect safety together tend to see desire return. That protection can look like longer arousal time before any insertion, liberal use of lubricant regardless of age, positions that allow the receiver to control depth and tempo, attention to pelvic floor relaxation, and medical or physiotherapy care when needed. Couples can decide that external pleasure will be the center for a season while comfort is rebuilt. Protecting association is the goal. Sex that is consistently safe teaches the body to approach again.

Long bonds sometimes confuse stability with sameness. Love holds, daily life functions, families grow, and erotic attention drifts because the brain adapts to predictable stimuli. Novelty that honors the relationship rather than threatening it can reawaken interest. You can change settings by moving to a different room or booking a low-stakes afternoon hotel rather than waiting for a once a year trip. You can change sequence by beginning with conversation about a shared memory, then kissing clothed, then showering, then alternating who receives. You can change pacing by setting a timer for ten minutes of one practice, such as only kissing or only oral, and promising not to rush. You can try a different sensory lead, such as music or scent, and see what that does to rhythm. This is not a quest for shock. It is the introduction of surprise small enough to feel safe and large enough to wake attention.

Attachment patterns show up in bed as clearly as they do in arguments. A person with anxious tendencies may search a partner's face for signs of rejection and lose arousal in the search. A person with avoidant tendencies may prefer to remain half clothed and half turned away, not because they do not care, but because exposure feels costly. Neither pattern is a flaw. Both require tenderness. The anxiously oriented partner often feels best when initiation includes explicit words of wanting that are not contingent on performance, and when aftercare includes reassurance that the connection remains secure regardless of how far a scene went. The avoidantly oriented partner often feels best when there is a plan that limits duration, predictable signals for pausing, and agreed moments of closeness that do not demand more closeness than they can tolerate. These small structures let both people relax.

Parents ask how any of this applies when privacy disappears and sleep runs thin. The answer looks ordinary. Locks on doors are health tools. Calendar holds count as foreplay. Trading childcare with friends once a month for two hours at home can matter more than a rare vacation. A movie for the children becomes a shower together that remains sensual even if no one reaches climax. Morning sex during cartoons can be sweeter than any complicated date night. The point is to treat erotic connection as part of family care rather than as a luxury you will get to someday.

Long distance couples develop their own art. Voice can carry more erotic power than images when used with care. One partner can read a short scene out loud during a call, including details that map to real bodies rather than fantasy bodies, then both can end with a promise about the next in-person visit. Texts can become breadcrumbs that tell a story over days without becoming pressure. Shared documents where partners write fantasies, boundaries, and aftercare wishes create a living map. Coordinated solo sessions that end with a brief debrief protect intimacy from becoming an abstraction.

Neurodivergent partners often benefit from higher explicitness. A written script for a scene can seem unromantic until you watch what happens to anxiety when guessing disappears. The script can list order, time boundaries, words that soothe, sensory preferences, and stop signals. Some autistic partners prefer low lighting, consistent rhythm, and limited eye contact during peak sensation, then deep eye contact during aftercare. Some partners with ADHD appreciate short, focused scenes early in the day and verbal cues that keep attention oriented to the body. None of this reduces passion. Clear structure makes room for it.

Disability and aging change technique without removing erotic capacity. Bodies that move differently can enjoy pressure and presence that do not depend on complex positions. Pillows become tools. Chairs become allies. Oral sex can replace penetration as the centerpiece without any loss of status. People with chronic illness often find that pain flares demand shorter scenes, more planning, and more gentleness afterward. Partners who learn to ask about pain levels, fatigue, and medication timing offer respect that reads as erotic because it communicates I want the real you, the one here today. Desire grows near that kind of regard.

Jealousy arrives in monogamous and nonmonogamous structures alike. In monogamy, jealousy often signals a need for more attention, more explicit wanting, or more reliability. Couples can answer it with shared rituals of reconnection, predictable intimacy windows, and repairs that do not leave loose ends. In consensual nonmonogamy, jealousy becomes information rather than accusation. Agreements about safer sex, testing schedules, disclosure pacing, and aftercare protect bonds. Some people imagine that new partners will fix a low desire pattern at home. Sometimes novelty briefly increases excitation. Often the underlying brakes remain, and they travel with you. No structure replaces the need to design context kindly.

Aftercare deserves a central place in partnered sex because it consolidates memory. A few minutes of holding, a glass of water, a snack, a warm cloth, a sentence about what worked, and a promise of next time, all of this tells the brain that the experience was complete and safe. After intense scenes, aftercare keeps the nervous system from interpreting the arousal peak as danger. After awkward scenes, aftercare prevents silence from writing a harsh story. Couples who treat aftercare as standard discover that trust deepens, and with trust comes willingness to take creative risks that make sex vivid again.

Repair after misses is how bonds remain erotic across time. You will move too fast one evening. You will freeze when you wished you had spoken. You will agree to something with your mouth while your body whispered a no. The next day contains a choice. You can ignore the miss and let your nervous systems file the memory under threat, or you can name what happened and propose a small adjustment. I realized I sped up when I felt you getting close, and I want to practice staying steady. I realized I agreed from obligation, and I want to try again when I can include myself. I realized I shut down when you touched my chest without warning, and I would like you to ask first. These lines are not confessions to a judge. They are instructions for the next scene.

Gratitude multiplies what works because it gives the giver a clear map. People sometimes assume appreciation is unnecessary. It is not. Say I loved the way you stayed with the same rhythm when my breath changed. Say When you asked whether I wanted more pressure, I felt cared for. Say The message you sent at lunch shifted my whole afternoon. Specific praise becomes a loop. The partner repeats the behavior because the nervous system loves reliable success, and both bodies get more of what they wanted.

Rejection requires ritual. No will occur, sometimes often, and without ritual a no can scrape the bond. The person declining can offer warmth and an alternate path. I am not available for penetration tonight, and I would love to kiss on the couch and hold you while you touch yourself, or I am a no now, and I am a yes tomorrow after coffee. The person hearing the no can respond in a way that keeps the door open. Thank you for telling me. I want to try again soon. When this dance becomes familiar, no stops meaning I do not want you and starts meaning I am caring for our bodies and our bond.

Weekly check-ins sound bureaucratic and function like relationship vitamins. Ten minutes on a Sunday morning can shift a month. Review one thing that worked last week and one thing to adjust. Pick one low stress window for intimacy and treat it as a plan rather than a wish. Mention any medical or parenting realities that change options. Ask small questions that lead to action. What would make you feel more wanted this week. What would make starting easier. When these short meetings become normal, erotic life no longer has to compete with logistics for attention.

There will be seasons when sex pauses or changes shape. Illness arrives, grief arrives, a newborn arrives, a new job swallows energy. Couples who remain erotic through those seasons do not pretend nothing changed. They agree on temporary frameworks that protect closeness. We will kiss every day even if our bodies are tired. We will lie naked together twice a week even if we nap instead of move. We will tell each other one fantasy sentence at bedtime even if we do not act on it. We will schedule a massage trade and let that count. These frameworks prevent long silences from hardening into distance.

If a relationship carries a history of hurt around sex, the path back begins with small, repeatable scenes that stay inside tolerance. Clothed back massage with clear stop signals is a classic for a reason. The giver practices patience. The receiver practices speaking in the middle of sensation. Then both debrief. I felt close when you asked permission to move lower. I felt scared when your hand sped up. Next time I want to say yellow sooner. These sessions build evidence that the room can be safe again, and evidence changes prediction more than promises ever could.

The thread that runs through every paragraph is agency shared. Partnered sex flourishes when both people feel their yes matters, their no will be honored, and their preferences are welcome as facts rather than as verdicts. It flourishes when the couple treats logistics as erotic because logistics shape safety. It flourishes when novelty is introduced with care. It flourishes when power is traded, gratitude is spoken, repair is common, and aftercare is standard. None of this requires perfect bodies or perfect timing. It requires attention, kindness, and practice.

Your relationship can carry two fully human nervous systems through decades if you treat sex as a living design problem rather than as a test. You will make a plan, you will try it, you will observe, you will adjust. You will keep context friendly to desire. You will remember that mismatched desire is a puzzle, not a diagnosis. You will let touch be generous and words be clear. When you do, partnered sex becomes easier to recognize as a place for play and comfort and adventure, all in the service of connection that fits the life you are actually living.

Chapter 10
Solo Sex, Fantasy, and Erotic Imagination

Private erotic life is a classroom, a studio, and a sanctuary. In the classroom you learn how your body responds, which rhythms gather intensity, which touches regulate a restless mind, which images open the door to desire. In the studio you practice, revise, and try again with patience that rarely survives in front of an audience. In the sanctuary you give yourself permission to feel pleasure without proving anything to anyone. When people reclaim this space as part of health, shame starts losing volunteers.

Many adults arrive with mixed feelings about masturbation. Some learned that it is childish, some learned that it signals relational failure, some learned that a "good" partner should not need it, and some learned, with a whisper, that it is fine as long as no one ever finds out. Those messages complicate a simple reality. Solo sex is a way to listen to your nervous system without pressure, to track the exact sequence that turns interest into arousal, and to build fluency you can bring back to a partner. If your culture of origin asked you to keep erotic life under lock and key, begin by renaming the practice. Call it rehearsal. Call it training. Call it care. Language shapes permission.

Pleasure benefits from preparation even when you are alone. Bodies carry the day inside them. If you want to shift from thinking to sensing, create a small ritual that does not depend on mood. You might silence notifications, dim a lamp, rinse your face, change into a soft T-shirt, and put a glass of water by the bed. None of this is fancy. What you are doing is telling your nervous system that the next twenty minutes have a single purpose. People who feel silly creating ambience for themselves often feel surprised when attention becomes easier the moment the room looks like it was prepared on purpose.

Arousal rises when the mind has a job. The most useful job is noticing, because noticing turns sensation into data you can use. At first you might slow your touch enough to describe it in words. This is a firm stroke along the outer labia. This is a steady circle just to the left of the glans. This is a squeeze that includes the shaft and the perineum. The sentences are not poetry. They are anchors. After a minute or two you can let the words fade and keep the attention. If thoughts wander toward errands or evaluation, return to breath. Inhale through the nose, exhale for a count that is longer than the inhale, keep the current rhythm of touch for several breaths before changing anything. Consistency lets the body climb rather than step down the ladder every thirty seconds.

Sequence matters, because many bodies do not want the most intense stimulation first. Start in wide circles and move inward slowly. Warm the skin before you focus. Notice which direction works best, which pressure makes the body unconscious of your hand and fully aware of the sensation. A lot of people think they should vary constantly to avoid boredom. Variation is helpful early. Later the system wants reliability. Once you feel the wave rising, keep everything the same for longer than seems reasonable. The reason orgasm can feel elusive for some is not a broken body. The reason is a pattern of adding novelty at the exact moment the nervous system is asking for repetition.

Fantasy supplies context when the room is quiet. There is a belief that fantasy must be spectacular. It does not. A single sentence can be enough. I am wanted here. I am in charge of the pace. I am safe to be slow and still be craved. I am allowed to be explicit. I am allowed to be tender. Some minds prefer a short scene with a setting, a door, a scent, and a sentence spoken at the right time. Some prefer a collage of sensations without faces. Some prefer memory. Some prefer invention. None of these choices betray a partner or a value, unless you decide they do. If an image conflicts with your ethics, identify which element carries the heat and rebuild a version that fits. If the charge is being chosen without hesitation, invite that ingredient into a story that also includes clarity and consent. You are teaching your brain to recruit motivation with material that does not injure conscience.

Imagination interacts with touch like a conversation. If fantasy outpaces sensation by too much, the body can feel left behind. If sensation leads without any story, attention can drift. Alternate leadership. Spend a minute following touch with a simple image, then pause the story and listen only to pressure and breath. If you notice that arousal spikes when a certain phrase enters your mind, memorize it. A line that works in private often works with a partner when softened into theme rather than script. I want you to choose me with words. I want you to tell me to slow down. I want you to praise me for staying present. Themes translate easily into action.

Toys deserve a place on the nightstand for the same reason we keep tools in the kitchen. Hands and mouths are versatile, yet they cannot deliver every frequency or shape. A small external vibrator can teach a clitoris how it likes to be approached, which helps a partner later. A sleeve can add compression and glide that a hand cannot sustain, which can be a relief to wrists and attention. A plug used gently with patience can make otherwise ordinary touch feel fuller because pelvic nerves share pathways. Hygiene and pacing matter. When exploring anal play alone, patience is protection. Use lubrication generously, breathe, and add increments so small they seem comical. Safety remains erotic when your body trusts you to stop the instant anything feels off.

People worry about training their bodies the "wrong" way. The fear is understandable, especially for those who enjoy quick, focused stimulation that partners rarely match. There is nothing wrong with quick releases. There is value in expanding repertoire. Plan sessions with different intentions. Some nights you sprint because stress needs a valve. Other nights you run long and slow, practice edging, and rest on the plateau without moving toward orgasm at all. The point is not virtue. The point is flexibility. Bodies that learn multiple paths arrive more easily even when conditions are not ideal.

Porn stands at the threshold of many private practices, which is why clarity helps. Visual erotic material can be arousing, efficient, and inspiring. It can also train expectations that do not fit your partner, your values, or your attention span. Agency is the test. If you can take breaks without distress, choose categories that align with your ethics, and use porn as one tool rather than the entire kit, you are in charge. If use becomes automatic, compulsive, or secret in ways that undermine intimacy, that is a signal to rebuild variety. Replace screens with erotic audio, fiction, or your own written scenes for a period. Notice whether arousal still rises. If it does not, you have found a place to train attention rather than a reason to shame yourself.

Religious and moral commitments deserve respect inside private life. You can hold a value that sex is sacred and still enjoy solo pleasure as preparation for ethical intimacy. You can hold a value about modesty and still learn your anatomy in detail so that you can communicate with honesty. You can hold a value of monogamy and still cultivate an imagination that keeps your bond fresh. Values and pleasure cooperate when the value is framed around care, consent, and integrity rather than control.

Trauma-aware solo practice is a path many survivors choose because it returns control to the person who lost it. Start far from genitals. Touch arms, shoulders, scalp, chest, thighs. Pair every transition with a spoken consent to yourself. I am choosing to move my hand to my belly. I can stop at any time. If images intrude, name that you are safe now. If dissociation arrives, pause and return to breath or a weighted blanket. You might set a timer for five minutes and deliberately end before overwhelm. The goal is not climax. The goal is association between sensation and safety. Over weeks or months that association can become strong enough that partnered touch no longer crosses the line from pleasure into threat.

Neurodivergent bodies thrive on structure. A checklist can look unromantic on paper and create more space for sensation in practice. The list might include room setup, the order of touch, the moment to introduce fantasy, the decision point for toys, and the plan for ending. Sensory preferences belong in writing. If bright light distracts, keep the lamp low. If certain fabrics irritate, keep a soft towel nearby. If eye contact disrupts concentration right before orgasm, allow yourself to look away. People with ADHD may prefer short, focused sessions earlier in the day and verbal cues that bring attention back to the body. Autistic partners often benefit from consistent rhythm and fewer surprises. None of these accommodations reduce intensity. They create the conditions in which intensity can arise.

Aging and disability change technique, not eligibility for pleasure. Hands that tire quickly can use tools that distribute effort. Joints that complain in certain positions can recruit pillows and chairs as allies. Numbness in one region can shift attention to another. People who live with chronic illness often discover that pacing matters more than ambition. Ten minutes of presence beats an hour of endurance. When the body has fewer green lights on a given day, the imagination becomes more important, and tenderness becomes more powerful.

Journaling after private practice teaches in ways memory cannot. You might write three sentences: what you tried, what intensified feeling, what softened it. Over time patterns appear. You learn that an inhale through the nose and a longer exhale helps more than changing hands. You learn that indirect clitoral touch for two minutes predicts better orgasm later than a direct start. You learn that firm pressure along the perineum in the last thirty seconds of a stroke can double your sense of fullness. You are building a manual for your own body. That manual becomes a love letter to anyone you invite close.

Some readers worry that solo sex will reduce interest in partnered sex. The data of lived experience usually says the opposite when secrecy and compulsion are not present. Private practice builds confidence and vocabulary. Confidence lowers anxiety. Lower anxiety increases access to pleasure with others. There are seasons when private life carries the weight because partnerships are complicated by illness, distance, conflict, or new parenthood. Solo pleasure during those seasons protects the erotic self from collapsing into dormancy and makes return easier when conditions improve.

Communication with partners about private practices can be a bridge rather than a wedge. You can say, I enjoy touching myself on days when we cannot be together, and it helps me stay connected to my body. You can say, I learned something last week about rhythm that I want to show you tonight. You can say, I prefer to keep some fantasy private, and I am happy to share themes that work for me. Agreements help. Decide whether porn appears in the relationship at all, and if so, when and how. Decide whether toys are introduced together or separately and whether some are shared. Decide how to signal a need for solo time without implying rejection. Transparency reduces fear, and reduced fear makes arousal more available.

When private life feels compulsive or flat, compassion is more useful than judgment. Compulsion often rides with loneliness, anxiety, or untreated depression. A flat landscape often rides with stress, medication effects, or pain. If you find yourself using intensity to outrun feeling or using frequency to manage numbness, recruit more support rather than harsher rules. Talk to a clinician about medication side effects. Seek therapy if past harm intrudes. Invite a friend to be an accountability witness if secrecy spirals. You are not weak for needing help. Erotic life is part of health, and health is communal.

Advanced play in private can look like mindfulness experiments rather than acrobatics. You might spend an entire session mapping the border between too much and not enough on the clitoral hood or the frenulum, taking notes about the smallest change that tips you into irritation or into loss of focus. You might practice starting with fantasy, then deliberately removing the story to see whether sensation now holds attention without narrative support, then reintroducing a gentle sentence to see if intensity jumps again. You might test breath as a dial, trying four-count inhale, six-count exhale, then five and seven, noticing which pattern carries you up the slope with the least muscle tension. None of this requires a stopwatch. Curiosity is the instrument.

Edging deserves more ink because it teaches patience and gives you options in bed with another person. Bring yourself to the edge where orgasm feels near, then soften pressure and breathe while maintaining the same location. Let the wave fall halfway, then rise again. If you prefer numbers, you can count breaths, two at the top and two at the plateau. If you prefer feel, you can wait for your pelvic floor to stop clenching before you climb again. The benefit shows up later when you can recognize the approach, ride it longer, and invite a partner to join you there without panic that the moment will evaporate if they do not move quickly enough.

The mind sometimes critiques the body in the middle of private play. Evaluation often sounds like a coach who never played. You took too long. You are boring. You are greedy. You are using fantasy wrong. Notice the voice and do not argue with it. Return to sensation. Evaluation feeds the brake. Attention feeds the accelerator. If the voice persists, give it a job no one wants. Ask it to count your breaths. Most inner critics grow sleepy when asked to do math.

People with a history of scrupulosity or moral anxiety can adapt the practice by borrowing rituals from spiritual life. Begin with a statement of intention. I am practicing pleasure as part of caring for a body I am responsible for. End with gratitude rather than apology. Thank you for the chance to feel good and to learn. Rituals reclaim solo sex from secrecy and align it with values that honor responsibility and kindness.

If you need to pause private practice for a while, do so without drama. Desire waxes and wanes in response to stress, grief, illness, medication, and fatigue. Pressuring yourself to perform solo sex on a schedule can turn the sanctuary into another task. Choose gentle engagement instead. You might rest with a hand on your chest and stomach, breathe in equal counts, and name one thing your body did for you today. That counts as erotic care because it keeps attention inside you. When you return to explicit touch, you will not feel like a stranger.

Body image sits in the corner of many rooms and comments on everything. If you hesitate to look at yourself, consider introducing sight gradually. Begin fully clothed and watch your face soften as you breathe. Watch your neck and your shoulders loosen. Later, choose clothing that feels kind and look at the places where sensation gathers. If you decide to be naked, meet your own eyes first. The goal is not immediate awe. The goal is familiarity. Bodies that are not looked at become imaginary bodies that never measure up to fantasy or to media. Real bodies, seen kindly, become eligible for joy.

Solo sex can support recovery from sexual pain by training relaxation rather than excitement. If penetration has hurt, private sessions can focus on external touch, on breath that lengthens exhale, on pelvic floor release rather than contraction, and on associations that pair arousal with comfort. A finger inserted only after long warm up, with abundant lubricant and zero pressure to continue, can be part of therapy. Dilators used with a focus on sensation and consent rather than on goals can help. When your body learns that your own hand will stop instantly, partners inherit that trust.

Long-distance seasons benefit from private skill. You can coordinate time with your partner, keep a voice call open, describe what you are doing in general terms, and agree to stop if anyone feels off. You can send each other short paragraphs that outline themes to try alone during the week, then debrief what worked. You can create shared playlists that cue breath and tempo. Private practice becomes a bridge rather than a substitute.

Parents, caregivers, and people with little privacy sometimes assume solo sex requires a perfect hour. It does not. Ten minutes with a locked door while children listen to an audiobook counts. Fifteen minutes in a bath with the shower running counts if the extra noise protects your mind from worry. Early mornings on a weekend count, even if you return to sleep immediately afterward. You are not selfish for using a lock. You are modeling boundaries in a house where everyone needs them.

If you want to integrate private discoveries into partnered scenes, start with the simplest transfer. Show a partner your preferred rhythm on your own body while they watch. Guide their hand with your hand and say less, more, slower, faster, stay. Bring a toy and demonstrate where it fits, then trade roles so they can feel what you felt. Name one theme from fantasy and translate it into two sentences that someone can say without acting. I want you here. I am with you. I like your sounds. I like your patience. Partners do not need to enter your inner theater. They need a cue they can carry.

The deepest payoff of private erotic life is not only stronger orgasms or a broader menu. The payoff is an internal relationship in which you treat yourself the way you want to be treated by others, with attention, curiosity, and respect. When you practice those qualities alone, you recognize them faster in relationships and you ask for them sooner. You also notice when they are missing. That feedback loops back into health, because sexual wellbeing is not a set of tricks. It is a way of being in your own body.

If you have read this far with a sense of permission growing, consider making a small promise to yourself. Choose one detail you will try this week. Maybe you will create a simple ritual for the room. Maybe you will write three lines of fantasy and read them out loud only to yourself. Maybe you will explore a toy without comparing your response to someone else's. Maybe you will practice edging for the first time, or for longer than usual, or not at all and rest on the plateau. Maybe you will keep a tiny log that records what worked and what did not, so that your future self inherits your knowledge. Whatever you choose, choose kindly.

Private erotic life belongs beside sleep, movement, and food as part of ordinary care. Treat it with the same steadiness. Some weeks it will be abundant, some weeks it will be quiet, some seasons it will carry you, some seasons it will ask to be carried. Keep listening. Keep learning. Keep translating what you learn into words you can say to someone who loves you. When solo practice and imagination become allies rather than secrets, desire stops feeling fragile and starts feeling like a resource you can cultivate, share, and enjoy across the changing landscape of your life.

Chapter 11
Sexual Pain, Trauma, and Pathways to Healing

Pain changes sex more quickly than almost anything else, because the nervous system learns fast when something hurts. One or two uncomfortable encounters can teach a body to anticipate harm. The lesson then repeats itself even in safer conditions, since prediction shapes sensation. People often blame desire for disappearing, when desire is doing exactly what it should do in the presence of threat. The task in this chapter is to name kinds of pain clearly, describe how trauma reshapes arousal and attention, and build practical pathways that restore safety first and pleasure next.

Begin with the facts many were never told out loud. Pain during sexual activity is common and treatable. There are medical reasons, muscular reasons, relational reasons, and historical reasons, which often overlap. A person can love their partner and still tense automatically when a hand moves toward the pelvis. A person can want closeness and still feel burning at the entrance of the vagina. A person can feel a deep ache with penetration because the cervix is being bumped, or sharp discomfort because the pelvic floor is contracting when it needs to relax. A penis owner can struggle with stinging during ejaculation from prostatitis, or experience curvature and soreness from Peyronie's disease, or feel pain because the foreskin does not retract comfortably. None of these experiences reduce worth or eligibility for intimacy. They are problems to be understood and treated.

Vulvas deserve precise language because precision reduces shame. When penetration burns at the entrance, especially with first contact, vestibulodynia may be present. The tissue around the vaginal opening can become sensitive for hormonal reasons, dermatologic reasons, chronic inflammation, or after a painful start to sexual life with a lot of bracing. Lubrication helps, yet lubrication alone does not solve tissue sensitivity. A clinician familiar with vulvar pain can evaluate for infections, dermatitis, hormonal change, and treat with topical medications, oral meds when appropriate, and referral to pelvic floor physical therapy. When pain sits deeper and feels like cramping or a pull on one side, endometriosis may be part of the picture. That pain often worsens with cycles, sometimes radiates to the back, and deserves gynecologic care that does not minimize symptoms. When the canal feels too tight to admit even a finger, when insertion triggers a reflexive closure, pelvic floor hypertonicity is likely. The words some clinicians still use, vaginismus or genito-pelvic pain and penetration disorder, describe a learned, protective contraction that can be unlearned with time, respect, and graded exposure.

Penises require the same honesty. Sharp pain with erection should be evaluated, because fibrous plaques in the tunica of the penis can change curvature and sensation. A foreskin that feels stuck or tears requires medical attention, not endurance. Burning with ejaculation may reflect infection or prostatitis. Anxiety can tighten muscles and reduce blood flow, which makes erections inconsistent and touch more irritating. Many men try to fight pain privately and interpret it as a failure of masculinity, then drift away from sex rather than ask for help. The better story says that sexual function belongs inside healthcare, and that relief rarely arrives through silence.

Trauma complicates the map by teaching the inhibition system to hold the brake hard. Sexual coercion, assault, intimate partner violence, childhood abuse, repeated pressure inside a relationship, homophobic or transphobic harassment, medical trauma during gynecologic or urologic procedures, shaming religious education, and painful childbirth experiences, all of these can leave traces that appear during erotic touch. Those traces take many forms. Some people feel numb and far away. Others feel flooded with images they did not invite. Others become incredibly polite and try to please while their bodies are shutting down. Others feel a sharp startle response when hands arrive without warning. The variation does not mean inconsistency. It means the nervous system found a way to protect the self in the moment harm was likely, and it has not yet received enough evidence to retire that job.

Understanding the biology helps because it removes blame. Pain and fear share pathways. The amygdala flags threat quickly. The insula tracks internal state and can magnify sensations once danger is predicted. The spinal cord can sensitize to repeated noxious input, which means later signals arrive louder even when the stimulus is mild. This is why a person who endured painful penetration for months can feel pain with a gentle attempt that would have been comfortable earlier in life. It is also why a person who endured ridicule or pressure can feel a wave of anxiety as soon as a scene begins, long before anything overtly sexual has happened. The body is not irrational. The body is efficient and conservative, built to prevent repeats of injury through caution.

Healing begins with safety that is real, observable, and practiced. A partner's patience matters more than any technique. The nervous system learns through repetition that boundaries will be honored immediately. Set agreements that are simple and enforceable. Ask before hands move toward genitals. Pause when the receiver says stop. Keep water nearby and offer it automatically after a pause. Stay with the person when they dissociate and speak in present-tense anchor statements. You are here with me in our room. Your feet are on the bed. You can breathe slowly and we will wait. These are not magic words. They are evidence delivered in real time that no one is going to push past a signal. Evidence creates new predictions. New predictions lower the brake.

Pelvic floor physical therapy deserves a full paragraph, because many people have never heard of it and it changes lives. The pelvic floor is a group of muscles that must coordinate relaxation and contraction for arousal, penetration, and orgasm. Chronic stress, guarding after pain, childbirth injuries, surgeries, and even posture habits can create patterns where these muscles stay clenched. A skilled therapist evaluates externally and internally with consent, teaches awareness of tension, guides release through breath and manual techniques, addresses alignment, and assigns home exercises that often include gentle stretching, internal massage with a gloved finger or a soft tool, and work with dilators. The word dilator frightens some people because they imagine force. In competent hands dilators are quiet tools used at the patient's pace, with generous lubrication, in tiny increments that the body chooses. Progress looks like a body that trusts entrance again, then begins to associate touch with comfort.

Medical care must be active and respectful. Persistent vulvar pain benefits from clinicians who understand that Q-tips do not diagnose character and that yeast cultures, dermatology consults, vestibular exams, and hormone discussions beat dismissive advice. Endometriosis requires providers willing to take pain seriously, try treatments stepwise, and refer for surgery when indicated. Prostatitis and pelvic pain in men benefit from urology and pelvic floor therapy together, not antibiotics forever. Peyronie's disease can be managed with physical therapy, medications, traction devices, or procedures when necessary. People assigned male at birth who learned to ignore foreskin pain deserve accurate information about options that preserve sensation and relieve tearing. People assigned female at birth who were told to endure dryness during hormonal transition deserve modern, safe local estrogen options discussed openly, along with moisturizers, lubricants, and time. In every case the doctor's posture matters. Patients who sense indifference or contempt often stop seeking help. Patients who sense curiosity and competence often heal faster simply because stress hormones recede in the exam room.

Psychotherapy that is trauma informed builds a bridge between body and meaning. Eye Movement Desensitization and Reprocessing can update traumatic memories so that images carry less charge. Somatic therapies teach interoception and help the person return to the present when old sensations surge. Cognitive work identifies shame beliefs that attach to sex and replaces them with language that honors values without punishing pleasure. Many survivors believe that pleasure makes them complicit with past harm, or that wanting makes them responsible for what happened. Therapy creates room for a more accurate map. The harm was the perpetrator's choice. Pleasure today, inside consent and care, belongs to the survivor.

Partners play a role that no clinician can play. They can choose a slower calendar and let intimacy rebuild in stages that preserve dignity. They can treat nonsexual contact as a valid endpoint rather than as a prelude that must always lead to penetration. They can narrate what their hands will do so that there are no surprises. They can ask what words soothe and what words trigger, then avoid the latter scrupulously. They can accept that some activities will be off the table for a season or forever, and they can show desire for the person rather than for a checklist. There is an art to wanting without pressure. It sounds like I want you in any way that feels good to you today. It looks like showing up for connection even when the menu is short. Bodies read that signal and often open sooner because the risk of letting someone close drops.

Graded exposure belongs in healing plans because the nervous system changes through small, repeated experiences under threshold. Start far from genitals with clothed touch that the receiver chooses and stops. Add breath, attention to warmth, and tiny doses of erotic language only when the body stays within tolerance. Move, over weeks, toward skin-to-skin contact, then to outer thighs and hips, then perhaps to the mons or pubic hair without moving lower. The process is slow compared to movie scenes and fast compared to the years many people have spent suffering. Each success writes a line of code in the brain. That line says this level of touch is safe. When enough lines accumulate, the system allows more.

Positions can prevent pain. Shallow angles protect a sensitive cervix. A receiver on top can control depth and tempo. Side-lying reduces pressure on the pelvic floor and low back. Pillows under hips can shift where penetration lands. Oral sex can replace penetration entirely without any loss of legitimacy. Hands and toys can deliver consistent pressure in places that feel good while avoiding places that do not. When couples treat technique as engineering rather than as a measure of passion, guilt fades and creativity grows.

Lubrication deserves zero apology. Natural moisture varies with arousal time, hydration, medications, cycles, and hormones. Generous lubricant reduces friction, prevents microtears, and allows slower pacing. Water-based products are easy to clean. Silicone-based products last longer and often help during menopausal dryness. Oil can disrupt condoms and some toys. If someone scoffs at lubricant, treat that as a script problem rather than a romance problem. Pleasure does not care about purity myths. Pleasure cares about comfort.

Pain flares during healing. Progress rarely moves in a straight line. A person can feel hopeful for two weeks and then experience a night that brings back fear. The right response to a flare is not to tighten rules or force a breakthrough. The right response is to shorten the scene, add aftercare, name triggers if they are visible, and plan a smaller step for next time. Many people overcorrect after a setback and declare the project a failure. Steady plans win. Short sessions that succeed consistently retrain the body faster than rare, ambitious attempts that overwhelm.

Religious and cultural trauma adds layers that deserve patient untangling. People who were told that sexual desire ruins purity may feel an immediate drop in arousal when they approach orgasm, as if a hand pulled a switch. People who were told that being desired is dangerous may dissociate the moment they feel seen. People who were told that pleasure is selfish may rush to end encounters as soon as their partner finishes and never receive. Spiritual counsel that honors consent and mutuality can help, as can therapy that separates inherited rules from chosen ethics. Many find it useful to write, in plain language, their adult sexual values, then compare those values to old lessons. The aim is not rejection of heritage. The aim is a translation that supports health.

Birth trauma lives in the pelvis and deserves mention wherever sexual pain is discussed. Tearing, scarring, changes in pelvic floor tone, and medical procedures performed without adequate explanation or analgesia can alter sensation for months or years. People often expect sexual function to return on a schedule that serves cultural narratives rather than healing. A more realistic plan gives time for tissue recovery, seeks pelvic floor therapy early, treats lactation-related dryness with moisture and local estrogen when appropriate, and reintroduces sexual touch slowly with full control in the postpartum parent. Partners can support by broadening definitions of intimacy during sleep-deprived months, by shouldering more household labor, and by refusing to treat the pelvis as public property after pregnancy.

Men carry pain and trauma too, though many were trained to hide it. A history of unwanted sexual experiences can produce erectile unpredictability that has nothing to do with attraction. Harsh comments about size or stamina can lodge in memory and trigger anxiety each time arousal begins. Prostate exams, catheterizations, and surgeries can leave behind hypervigilance during anal or perineal touch. Treatment looks similar regardless of gender. Slow exposure, attention to consent, therapy when memories intrude, medical care for tissue causes, and partners who distinguish between performance and presence.

Communication remains the spine of every plan. Couples who heal well talk in short sentences during scenes and longer sentences on off days. In the moment they say softer, slower, stay there, lower, stop, start again, I am with you. On off days they say when you asked before moving your hand, I felt safe, or I noticed a surge of fear when I lost your face for a second, or I want to try side-lying next time with a pillow and no goal beyond warmth. This specificity prevents guessing and keeps shame from filling gaps.

Aftercare is medicine. Bodies need help shifting from high arousal or high vigilance back to baseline. A warm cloth, a glass of water, a snack, a few minutes of quiet holding, a brief review of what worked, and a plan for the next attempt, all of this tells the nervous system that the story ended well. After intense scenes, aftercare also prevents the brain from mislabeling the experience as stress. Couples who treat aftercare as standard report faster progress and fewer spirals of misinterpretation.

Self-compassion speeds healing more than grit ever did. Many people believe they must push through pain to prove strength. The data says otherwise. Bodies that feel respected reduce protective responses. People who speak to themselves as they would to a friend recover attention to pleasure sooner. If you hear an inner voice say you are too much work, answer with a sentence you would give a loved one. I am learning, I am allowed to go slowly, I am worth this care. The words may feel mechanical at first. Repetition turns them into a baseline.

Measure progress in practical units. A month ago you could not tolerate a hand resting over clothing on the hips for more than thirty seconds. Today you stayed with it for three minutes and your breath remained even. Two weeks ago deep penetration hurt immediately. Today, with a pillow and slower pace, you felt comfortable for a short time and stopped before pain started. Last season you dissociated during kissing when surprised. This week your partner asked each time and you stayed present for the whole kiss. These are not small wins. They are the bricks that rebuild erotic confidence.

Invite community where it helps. A knowledgeable clinician, a pelvic floor therapist, a sex therapist, and a supportive friend can form a quiet circle around your process. Groups for survivors of sexual assault or for people with chronic pelvic pain can normalize the path and reduce loneliness. Books, podcasts, and educators who use accurate language can replace myths with maps. Privacy remains your right. Isolation is not required.

If substance use became part of coping with sexual fear or pain, healing can include new ways to regulate. Many people drink to reduce vigilance. Unfortunately alcohol dulls sensation and can increase pain later. Breath practices, warm baths, slow stretches, laughter that loosens the jaw and shoulders, and predictable scripts for initiation give the same nervous system relief without dulling the very signals you need to hear while you relearn comfort.

A note for partners who want to help and feel lost. Your job is not to fix. Your job is to make it easy for your loved one to set the pace, to celebrate small successes, to accept pauses with grace, and to bring desire to the version of intimacy that is possible today. Some partners grow anxious when sex changes shape and pull away to avoid doing harm. Pulling away can feel like rejection. Stay close in the ways that are welcome. Hold hands during television. Send a message at lunch that says you are wanted. Ask what day this week would feel easiest for a small scene. Attend appointments when invited. Your reliability is medicine.

For readers whose pain has lasted years and who fear that pleasure has moved out permanently, consider a compact you make with yourself today. The compact says that you will seek competent care, that you will not accept dismissal, that you will practice one small thing three times a week for eight weeks, that you will measure progress in comfort and presence rather than in number of orgasms, and that you will protect your body from any activity that forces it to perform. Eight weeks of steady, kind practice often moves what years of avoidance do not.

Eventually the goal shifts from the absence of pain to the presence of pleasure. That shift arrives quietly. One evening you notice warmth spreading without worry. One morning you feel arousal return as soon as a partner says the sentence that always steadies you. One day you realize that your body did not flinch when a hand moved along its old path. Healing never asks you to forget. Healing asks you to tell a new truth that sits beside the old one. This touch is safe. This room honors me. This partner listens. My body can learn again.

Sexual wellbeing includes the right to comfort and the right to joy. You do not need to earn those rights by enduring harm. You do not need to prove toughness by ignoring pain. You can decide that your pelvis deserves the same careful attention you give to your heart or your lungs. You can collect a team, change a script, ask for a slower pace, choose positions that protect you, and close scenes with care. With time the nervous system recalculates. It begins to predict pleasure where it once predicted danger. That recalculation is the doorway back to the erotic life you deserve.

Chapter 12
Sexuality Across the Lifespan

Bodies never stop changing, and erotic life changes with them. If you try to hold sex still while everything else moves, frustration will follow. A wiser approach treats sexuality as a living practice that adapts to seasons, learns from history, and welcomes new capacities as they arrive. That frame turns aging from a threat into a teacher. It also protects younger readers from thinking they must peak by a certain age to be legitimate. There is no single prime. There are many primes, each with its own pleasures and skills.

Childhood sets the foundation long before desire appears. The way adults respond to curiosity about bodies plants early scripts that either support consent or undermine it. A child who hears accurate words for vulva, penis, anus, and chest learns that the body can be spoken about without shame. A child who is allowed to say no to hugs learns that boundaries persist even with family. A child who sees caregivers repair after conflict learns that closeness and safety can coexist. These lessons are not sexual in the adult sense. They are relational habits that will later shape how that person gives and receives pleasure.

Puberty arrives with speed and confusion. The brain retools attention, reward, and social sensitivity at the same time that hormones transform skin, hair, sweat, and genitals. Many teenagers feel like they are driving a new vehicle at night without headlights on unfamiliar roads. What helps is straightforward information framed around respect: how erections, lubrication, and orgasm work; how consent sounds; how contraception and safer sex are obtained; how porn is performance rather than instruction; how social media amplifies comparison.

Adults often worry that honest education invites behavior. In practice, secrecy invites risk. Teens who know how to protect themselves and how to say no also know how to seek care when something goes wrong.

First partnerships tend to magnify everything. Novelty is high, insecurities are loud, and the wish to be good becomes a kind of test. Many young adults imagine that technique will compensate for anxiety. Bodies seldom cooperate with that plan. What usually works better is pacing and honesty. A partner who says, I am new to this and want to learn, makes the room safer for both people. A partner who says, I need to move slower than movies suggest, prevents pressure from writing the first chapter. These early scenes often carry more influence than people realize. When they are kind, the memory system learns that erotic life is a place of curiosity. When they are rushed or humiliating, the memory system grows watchful and presses the brake.

Queer and trans youth navigate an extra labyrinth. Attraction that does not match family expectation can produce secrecy and fear. Gender dysphoria can make arousal feel like betrayal when the body responds in ways that do not reflect identity. Supportive adults become lifelines. A simple sentence like, your experience is real and you deserve comfort and respect, can dilute shame better than any lecture. Access to gender-affirming care changes erotic life as well as mental health. When a person recognizes themselves in the mirror, they can include their body in pleasure instead of dissociating from it.

Early adulthood usually offers the most novelty a person will ever see. New partners, new apartments, new jobs, and new freedoms create opportunity and overwhelm. Many people experiment with relationship structures, from monogamy to consensual nonmonogamy, and discover that agreements matter more than labels. Some chase intensity and misinterpret stimulus overload as proof of compatibility. Some avoid conflict and interpret silence as peace. Erotic maturity in this decade often means learning to match values with actions. If you want caring sex, choose partners who care. If you want reliability, choose partners who repair. The principle sounds simple and becomes profound once you start using it.

Contraception, fertility, and pregnancy enter the conversation for many people next. Desire fluctuates across menstrual cycles, often rising near ovulation and falling during certain premenstrual days. Hormonal contraception can decrease libido in a subset of users, and for others it reduces anxiety about pregnancy enough to increase desire. The only reliable rule is to listen to the body you have and adjust context accordingly. Pregnancy can bring increased blood flow and sensitivity for some, fatigue and nausea for others. Many couples find that sex during pregnancy becomes more creative as positions change to respect comfort and as penetration yields some nights to external pleasure. Perinatal care that mentions sexuality as a normal part of health helps parents return to erotic life without feeling that the pelvis has become public property.

Postpartum months alter almost everything at once. Sleep fragments, bodies heal, attention narrows to a new person who arrives with needs that ignore the clock. Estrogen drops, which can reduce lubrication, while oxytocin rises, which can increase bonding and reduce social threat. Some parents feel sexual interest disappear and fear it will never return. Others feel desire soften into a wish for closeness without intensity. What works is patience plus design. Protect naps, share the mental load, use generous lubricant, and redefine success as connection rather than climax. The parent who did not give birth can initiate care rather than sex, can handle tasks without prompting, and can praise the other's body for its strength rather than for its similarity to its past form. Erotic life returns more quickly when no one pressures it to perform on a schedule that serves a timeline rather than a family.

The thirties and forties often bring career demands, caregiving for aging relatives, and the arithmetic of time. Stress is high, novelty is low, and many couples mistake the absence of spontaneous desire for loss of love. Responsive desire becomes common in these years. It shows up after touch begins, not before. Couples who accept that pattern adjust initiation and add deliberate warm up on nonsexual days. Scheduling intimacy begins to look less like bureaucracy and more like respect for the nervous system. Medical realities appear too. Antidepressants can delay orgasm. Blood pressure medication can affect erection. Attention conditions like ADHD can make sustained focus difficult. None of this removes the possibility of satisfying sex. It invites conversations that include detail: longer runway, consistent rhythm, earlier windows, more external stimulation, and a wider definition of what counts.

Perimenopause enters for many people with ovaries in the forties, sometimes earlier. Estrogen levels fluctuate, cycles change, sleep becomes less reliable, and mood may move through wider ranges. Genital tissue may feel thinner and drier. The cultural story often predicts decline. A better story predicts adjustment. Local vaginal estrogen restores elasticity and lubrication safely for most. Silicone lubricant lasts longer. Longer warm up gives blood flow time to arrive. Many discover that explicit communication becomes easier in midlife because there is less interest in pretending. That ease opens doors. Some women report that once reproductive vigilance recedes, pleasure becomes more accessible because the body is no longer scanning for pregnancy risk. Others discover that external stimulation now outperforms penetration, and they reorganize sex accordingly. A partner who treats these changes as upgrades rather than losses helps the system move without shame.

People with testes face their own midlife transitions. The phrase andropause is imprecise, yet many men notice slower arousal, less reliable morning erections, and a need for more direct stimulation. Some panic and interpret the change as a verdict on masculinity. Panic increases performance anxiety, which makes erection less reliable. The better approach uses engineering and kindness. Extend warm up, use a sleeve or a vibrator as part of shared play, shift attention from penetration as the only proof of sex to multiple routes of giving and receiving pleasure, and consult a clinician about cardiovascular health, hormones, and medications. Erections are vascular events. A checkup that protects the heart also protects the penis.

Divorce and repartnering often occur in these decades. People return to dating with bodies that carry histories, and the scripts of early adulthood no longer fit. Safety requires more conversation now. Testing, contraception, and boundaries deserve explicit language before bodies meet. Widowed and divorced adults often feel shy about reentering sexual culture. Tenderness solves shyness. You can say, I am excited and nervous. I want to go slowly and talk a lot. You can say, I need to stop and check in sometimes because my body learns new people through caution. Partners who welcome that pace are partners worth keeping.

Menopause arrives eventually and rewrites the hormonal landscape permanently. Estrogen remains low, which affects vaginal tissue and urinary tract health. Testosterone, present in all bodies, can also shift. Some women experience a dip in libido; others feel steady or even freer. Pleasure remains possible at any level of hormones. What changes are the inputs required. Regular local estrogen, moisturizers, and high-quality lubricant protect tissue. Strength and flexibility work protect joints and back during favorite positions. Attention to pelvic floor health prevents pain. Many couples discover that sex slows down in a way that deepens presence. The speed of youth is replaced by a steadier rhythm that allows longer savoring. There is grief in change and there is gain.

Aging past sixty exposes myths. One myth says older adults have no sexual interest. Another says that erectile changes or lubrication changes end intimacy. Reality is kinder and more diverse. Many older adults report high satisfaction when they adapt. Some have frequent intercourse. Some shift to external focus. Some keep sex softer on most nights and reserve intensity for special windows. Many report an increase in body gratitude, a decrease in self-consciousness, and an appetite for affection and erotic warmth that feels more central than any single act. Medical settings sometimes ignore this part of life. Patients can insist. Ask your clinician about medication side effects, about local estrogen, about PDE5 inhibitors and cardiovascular screening, about pelvic floor therapy. Health systems will change faster when patients ask loudly.

STI prevention belongs at every age. Older adults who reenter dating may not see themselves in safer-sex campaigns and may underestimate risk. Condoms, dental dams, testing, and honest disclosure protect everyone without reducing romance. A conversation that begins with, I want this to go well for both of us, so let's plan for safety, often increases trust. Trust increases arousal. The equation remains the same regardless of decade.

Disability intersects with sexuality across the lifespan in ways that textbooks rarely cover. Conditions that alter mobility, sensation, stamina, or pain tolerance require creativity, not resignation. People with spinal cord injuries can experience orgasm through pathways that bypass the injury, including vagus-mediated routes. People with chronic pain can enjoy shorter scenes that respect flare patterns, with longer aftercare that prevents rebound discomfort. People who use wheelchairs can explore positions that recruit chairs as allies. Adaptive toys and pillows can transform access. Partners who ask, what works today, and mean it, create a present-focused erotic culture in the relationship that resists despair.

Neurodivergence travels with people from childhood to old age, and it shapes erotic life politely when honored. Autistic adults may prefer steady rhythm, predictable order of operations, and no sudden transitions. Adults with ADHD may prefer brief, intense sessions earlier in the day and more verbal anchors to keep attention inside sensation. Sensory processing differences can make certain fabrics, scents, or pressures uncomfortable or intensely pleasurable. Self knowledge and scripts protect dignity. People who learn to say, Here is what makes my body cooperate, arrive in midlife with an erotic language that many neurotypical couples only discover after years of guessing.

Religious and cultural identities evolve across decades and influence sex at every step. A person who spent youth in purity culture may choose in midlife to keep commitments to fidelity and care while releasing rules that punished desire. Another may discover at seventy that queerness has always been present and deserves daylight now. Communities respond with a range of grace. The internal anchor remains the same: health is congruence between values and behavior, and values centered on dignity, consent, and mutuality support erotic life from adolescence to elderhood.

Grief visits many beds across time. Illness, miscarriage, infertility, abortion, disability, divorce, and death change bodies and relationships. Sex can pause, morph, or become a place of comfort. There is no correct response. What protects couples is permission to let erotic life take the form that matches the season. Sometimes that form is holding each other while tears come. Sometimes it is laughing in bed at how wildly unsexy life has been and finding small sparks again. Sometimes it is a sabbatical with dates on the calendar for review so that pause does not become a silence that no one knows how to break.

Caregiving is a late-life theme that many never imagined when they said vows or chose a partner. Dementia, stroke, cancer, and chronic illness recruit partners into roles that mix devotion with exhaustion. Consent becomes complex when cognition changes. Intimacy may need to shift toward touch that is affectionate rather than erotic, toward routines that soothe rather than excite, toward rituals that preserve mutual dignity. Caregivers deserve erotic care for themselves as well, whether through solo practice, therapy to metabolize grief, or time with friends who remember them as more than a role. Sexual health widens here to include the health of the person doing the caring.

Throughout all decades, fantasies evolve. A person who once needed novelty may discover that reverence now works better. A person who once needed control may find deep arousal in being guided. A person who once avoided eye contact may find that gaze becomes the center of sex at seventy. Themes stay, characters change. The permission to update is a gift you can give yourself repeatedly. Eroticism is less about age than about attention and kindness inside the age you are.

Practical guidance helps when theory runs long. At every stage ask three questions. What does my body need more of to feel safe and engaged. What does it need less of to stop bracing. What meanings encourage me to show up. In adolescence the answers might be accurate information, less secrecy, and the belief that I am allowed to say no. In the thirties the answers might be sleep, fewer late-night attempts, and the belief that responsive desire is normal. In menopause the answers might be local estrogen, less rushing, and the belief that pleasure still belongs to me. In the eighties the answers might be gentle pressure, less performance anxiety, and the belief that bodies at any age deserve to be cherished.

Partnerships survive change when they treat sexuality as a shared design project. You and your partner will revisit agreements as bodies heal, tire, and awaken. You will decide to schedule more and guess less. You will agree that external stimulation counts as complete. You will decide that mornings work better now. You will create new initiation signals when the old ones feel confusing. You will protect aftercare as standard. You will forgive misses more quickly because you both understand the forces you are facing. Couples who adopt this stance in their twenties are grateful for it in their seventies.

For readers traveling alone, the same design principle applies. Solo practice keeps the erotic self alive during seasons without partnership and teaches skills you bring back when partnership returns. The belief that private pleasure is a placeholder belongs to a culture that prizes performance over presence. Private pleasure is a practice in listening. People who keep listening across decades tend to build relationships that respect their bodies because they already respect themselves.

Let this chapter end with portraits rather than prescriptions. Picture a woman in her late fifties who schedules a pelvic floor consultation, buys two kinds of lube, asks her doctor about local estrogen, and then plans three afternoons with her partner to try positions that protect her back, laughing each time they slide off the pillows. Picture a man in his sixties who feels ashamed of slower erections, tells his partner the truth, extends warm up, adds a toy that both enjoy, and discovers that orgasms feel richer because the scene slowed down enough for his mind to arrive. Picture a nonbinary person in their twenties who finds a therapist, learns to negotiate touch that affirms their gender, and uses fantasy to build a sense of being chosen in the exact body they live in. Picture a lesbian couple in their seventies who meet every Sunday to plan the week, mark one afternoon for intimacy, and count a two-hour session of sensual massage as a success whether or not anyone climaxes. Picture a widower who thought erotic life was over, practices gentle solo touch, joins a group at the community center, and one day accepts coffee with someone who speaks kindly, then months later discovers that his body knows how to feel alive with another person again.

Across the lifespan, sexuality thrives where people update expectations, protect safety, and keep curiosity. You can be newly brave at sixteen or at sixty. You can learn to speak clearly as a teenager or as a grandparent. You can shift techniques because hormones shifted. You can ask for what fits the body you have instead of chasing the body you once had. You can love with tenderness and play in every decade available to you. If you remember nothing else, remember this: erotic life is not a race to a vanishing finish line. It is a conversation that grows wiser every time you return to it.

Chapter 13
Digital Intimacy: Porn, Sexting, Apps, and Consent Online

Phones live beside our beds, in our pockets, on the table where we eat. Sexuality has moved into those same spaces, quietly and completely. Desire now meets push notifications, algorithms, high-definition video, encrypted chats, dating feeds, and private archives of photos that can travel across the world in a heartbeat. For some readers this new terrain feels liberating. For others it feels like a maze filled with bright rooms and hidden trapdoors. A healthy digital erotic life asks the same questions you ask about sex in person. Am I safe. Do I have agency. Do I know what I want from this experience. Can I stop. Will my choices today help the person I am becoming. Those questions guide you better than any single rule.

Pornography sits at the center of most conversations about sex and the internet, so begin there with clarity instead of panic. Visual erotic material can be arousing, informative, and efficient, and it can also create friction with values, attention, or relationships when it replaces variety or when secrecy grows. The human visual system is sensitive to motion, novelty, and faces. Video therefore recruits attention quickly, often faster than imagination or touch. Algorithms learn what you pause on and deliver more of it. That pairing of biology and machine learning can feel like momentum that carries you farther than you intended. The antidote is not shame. The antidote is agency. Decide in advance what role porn plays in your life, which categories match your ethics, how often you want to use it, whether you prefer solo use or shared use, and how you will intervene when use begins to feel automatic rather than chosen.

Couples benefit from explicit agreements because assumptions break easily in digital spaces. Two partners can love each other and imagine very different rules. One may think private viewing is fine if the content is legal and consensual and if attention returns to the relationship afterward. The other may feel excluded by secrecy even if the content itself is mild. A workable conversation sounds like this. I want to understand what porn does for you, and I want to tell you what happens in my body when I know you used it. Then you trade specifics. I notice that when I watch in the afternoon I arrive at night already less present. I notice that when I find out after the fact I feel like a substitute rather than a partner. Together you design guardrails. Some couples choose categories that fit shared values and watch together occasionally, then reserve other nights for touch without screens. Some choose solo use with disclosure once a week in two sentences. Some choose to pause entirely for a month and rebuild erotic variety with imagination and speech. None of these choices proves virtue. They simply align behavior with what the relationship can hold.

Claims about addiction appear in many headlines and deserve careful language. People can absolutely develop patterns of use that feel compulsive, that crowd out other activities, that blunt arousal with partners, or that conflict with values. Those patterns respond best to the same strategies that help with any behavior that has become sticky. Increase variety so that excitement does not depend on one pathway. Introduce friction by moving devices out of the bedroom at night or by setting app limits you must actively override. Replace high-intensity scrolling with slower erotica in audio or text when your goal is presence rather than speed. Ask what feelings the behavior manages. Loneliness, anxiety, and shame often sit underneath.

Treat the feeling, not only the habit. If the pattern continues to run you, recruit help from a clinician who understands sexual behavior without moral panic, and involve your partner in a plan that includes both of your needs.

Ethics matter because bodies on screens belong to people. Choose sources that verify consent, age, and working conditions. Pay for what you use if you want a landscape where creators can set boundaries and refuse coercion. Avoid material that trades on intoxication, humiliation without negotiation, or racialized stereotypes presented as entertainment. If you would be ashamed to summarize the scenario to a friend you respect, your body is telling you something about alignment. People often believe that ethics dampen arousal. In practice, ethics remove background noise so that arousal can rise without conflict.

Sexting looks simple from the outside and becomes delicate the moment you involve names, faces, and metadata. A private photo feels intimate because it is. You are trusting someone with an image that can be copied endlessly. Before you send the first picture, decide your boundaries in daylight. What parts of your body will you show. What identifiers will you keep out of frame. What happens to the images if the relationship changes. How will you store or delete the thread. You can write a small agreement together. We send images only when asked and when sober. We do not forward or screenshot. If the relationship ends, we both delete within twenty-four hours and confirm in writing. People sometimes roll their eyes at formality, until a friendship ends or a breakup hurts and a simple clause protects dignity.

Style helps with both safety and arousal. Cropping faces reduces risk without removing heat. Clothing, shadows, and angles can be far more erotic than explicit exposure because suggestion invites imagination. Captions can carry more charge than pixels when they speak to the exact dynamic you share. I am thinking about your hand at the back of my neck. I am leaving work early and want your mouth on my shoulder before we talk. I want to be told to slow down and breathe while you watch. These sentences travel safely where pictures cannot.

Risk does not come only from partners. Laws in many places treat nude images of minors as contraband even when the images were created by the minor, and penalties can be catastrophic. Parents and teens need straightforward guidance. Do not create or store sexual images of yourself or anyone else under the age of consent. If someone sends you such an image, do not save or forward. Delete, block, and tell a trusted adult. Adults have their own legal risks. Workplace policies, school codes, and professional standards can interpret private conduct broadly. Convenience rarely protects you. Delay gratification long enough to ask whether the context is safe.

Image-based abuse, sometimes called nonconsensual pornography, requires words that match the harm. A private photo shared without permission is not gossip. It is a violation. Survivors deserve immediate care, not lectures. If this happens to you, you can collect evidence with screenshots and timestamps, contact platforms through their reporting tools for intimate image abuse, involve a lawyer or advocate when possible, and ask friends to help chase copies so that you are not alone in the grind. Many jurisdictions now recognize this harm in law. Even when legal systems move slowly, social systems can respond quickly. Communities that treat confidentiality as sacred reduce the secondary trauma that often follows exposure.

Dating apps are the new town square. Profiles act like billboards for selves that are edited to fit small screens, and swipes give the illusion of infinite choice. Underneath the game sits a set of ordinary human problems. People want to be seen and to belong. People want novelty and safety at the same time. People want chemistry and reliability in the same person. Apps can help when you treat them as introductions rather than as verdicts on your worth. A clear profile does more than list preferences. It teaches potential partners how to succeed with you. Say what you are available for in simple terms. Interested in a relationship that includes affection in public, laughter, and honest sex talks. Allergic to ghosting. Turned on by kindness and a plan. If you prefer something casual, you can still be humane. Looking for connection that can be playful and warm. Prefer texting less and seeing each other more. Care about consent and clarity. This tone reduces mismatches.

First conversations serve as miniature laboratories. Does the other person ask questions or perform monologues. Do they respect small boundaries, like waiting for your reply rather than sending six messages in a row. Do they use sexual language that matches your pace, or do they press for explicit material before trust exists. When someone moves too fast, you can slow the dance without dramatics. I prefer to meet before we trade anything intimate. If that boundary is welcomed, interest has room to grow. If it is mocked or ignored, the app saved you weeks.

Consent online operates by the same principles as consent in person, yet it needs more checks because asynchronous communication removes body cues. Ask before sending explicit material. Wait for clear yes. Track tone rather than content alone. A positive message written with fear or pressure behind it deserves a pause. Treat silence as no. Build in check-ins. Do you want more of this. Would you like a photo or a call or neither. Tell me to stop if I miss the mark. People worry that questions will kill the spark. Over time the opposite usually occurs. Questions teach both of you that desire is welcome and that boundaries hold. Boundaries raise desire because they lower vigilance.

Long-distance relationships live and die by digital practice. Many survive years because they design ritual rather than default to longing. Schedule regular video dates with themes. Cook the same meal in separate kitchens, then eat together while telling each other a memory no one else knows. Choose a night for reading out loud, which lets voice do what hands cannot. Send a short voice note before sleep that names one detail you loved about the other person this week. Plan coordinated solo scenes sometimes and end with aftercare on the phone so that the body receives closure. Agree on how to handle jealousy and loneliness before they bite. A sentence like I am feeling the emptiness tonight and need extra messages can prevent a fight that would have been about distance rather than about character.

Virtual reality and interactive toys promise immersion. For some couples these tools bridge touch across miles. For others they feel uncanny or invasive. The same rule applies. Decide the role they will play rather than letting the device decide for you. If you try VR, set a time boundary and debrief after the scene. What felt more present. What felt less human. If you integrate app-connected toys, agree on who controls them and when. One partner can bring a device to a work trip and give the other scheduled windows to play, then both can talk afterward about how power, surprise, and distance felt. Novelty serves intimacy when it follows consent.

Creators, sex workers, and subscription platforms occupy a growing slice of digital erotic life. Some readers create content. Some subscribe to it. Some do both. Respect means using the same ethics you bring to any marketplace where bodies are central. Do not pirate. Do not pressure. Do not imagine relationship where a transaction lives, and do not deny the humanity of a person who makes erotic labor their craft. If you are partnered and choose to subscribe, include that in your agreements. Your partner may feel less threatened when your choices are named, bounded, and connected to your shared values.

Performance anxiety has learned a new costume in the age of endless content. People compare themselves not only to exes or friends, but to edited montages staged by professionals. The comparison then creeps into bed. A partner tries to perform a scene rather than to feel. A receiver tries to react with the speed or intensity of a clip. Bodies notice the mismatch and shut down. The way back to sensation is boring on paper and powerful in practice. Close screens for a season. Replace visual speed with spoken fantasy that belongs only to the two of you. Recover patience by staying with one rhythm long enough to feel its effect instead of chasing five thrills in five minutes. Speak appreciation out loud so that the body hears you are here rather than you are being measured against an invisible standard.

Privacy has become a health behavior. Your phone contains an erotic archive even if you never meant to build one. Messages, photos, search histories, app data, cloud backups, and notification previews act like little windows into your interior life. Protecting those windows protects your relationships and your future self. Use a screen lock. Turn off previews on the lock screen. Separate work devices from personal ones where possible. Store intimate media in an encrypted vault rather than in the camera roll. Back up carefully if you must, and never automatically to shared albums. Say out loud to a partner how you plan to protect their images. The sentence I keep your photos in a locked folder and I never back them up to the cloud may sound technical. It reads as love.

Data collected by sex tech companies deserves attention because it often includes sexual orientation, device usage, and even physiological metrics. Before you connect a toy to an app, read what the company collects and whether they sell or share that information. Choose products that store data locally or that let you opt out. People sometimes protest that they have nothing to hide. The argument misses the point. Intimacy belongs to you. Handing it to strangers does not make sex freer. It makes sex marketable. You are allowed to keep what is yours.

Communities grow online where they rarely survive offline. Kink educators host classes. Asexual forums create language for lives that were ignored. Trans creators share practical advice about dysphoria, hormones, and pleasure. Survivors organize for safety and care. The internet multiplies your chances of finding people who share your needs and values. Participation stays healthy when you remember that avatars hide context. A kind teacher might be terrible fit for you. A person who types with certainty might be twenty and guessing. Take what helps, give credit, and keep your pace.

Jealousy changes shape when desire meets feeds. A partner may feel a sting when they see what you like or who you follow. The sting sometimes hides a simple request. Please want me out loud, not only other people on a screen. You can answer that request without deleting your interests. Tell your partner in words what you love about their body. Send a private message that says I am thinking about your mouth later, not only to a public account that will never reply. The algorithm will not care how you feel. Your relationship will.

People ask whether digital life ruins sex. The better question asks what kind of digital life supports the sex you want. If your goal is warmth and presence, keep your phone off the bed and your voice in the room. If your goal is exploration, choose creators and communities that align with your ethics and leave you feeling more connected rather than more depleted. If your goal is to keep desire alive across distance or time, use technology to deliver anticipation rather than constant noise. The device is a tool. You are the user.

Practical scripts help when you feel shy. Before sending a photo you can write I want to share something intimate. Are you in a place where that feels good to receive. Before asking for a photo you can write I love the way you look when you wake up. Would you send me a picture in that T-shirt. If someone sends something you did not ask for, you can write I am not available for explicit images without agreement. Please check first. If a partner's viewing habits unsettle you, you can say I want to understand what you watch and how it lands in your body. I also want to tell you why some of it sits wrong for me. Can we design a plan that protects both of us. If an app conversation turns sexual too fast, you can say I prefer to meet before we go there. If that timing does not work for you, I wish you well.

Education for young people needs to name the online world or it will arrive anyway without guidance. Adults can say, directly and calmly, that porn exists to entertain, that actors rehearse, that scenes are edited, that consent in real life is messy and ongoing, that bodies vary, that lubricant and communication matter, that images on phones can harm reputations and relationships, that no one has the right to your photos, and that you can always come home if something goes wrong. Young people who hear accurate words from trusted adults are more likely to speak up when they need help.

Faith communities and cultural groups have a role to play here as well. Values framed around dignity, consent, honesty, fidelity where promised, and care for vulnerable people can guide digital choices without denying desire. Congregations and community centers can host workshops on online safety and intimacy. Youth leaders can learn how to answer questions without shaming bodies. Elders can tell the truth about how intimacy changes with age, including how technology helped or hurt. Silence cedes the ground to algorithms.

If you work in a profession that depends on public trust, you carry risks that deserve extra caution. Teachers, physicians, therapists, clergy, public officials, and others often face policies that treat private conduct broadly. Assume that anything you create could travel. This does not mean you must live without erotic privacy. It means your privacy practices must be strict, your partners must be trustworthy, and your boundaries must be clear. You can design an erotic life that keeps your vocation intact.

Relationships end. Digital traces linger. Plan your endings with the same care as your beginnings. Delete shared folders. Remove access to smart devices. Return or destroy toys that hold data. Close joint subscriptions. Clear chats with a brief, kind message that says I am deleting our thread to give us both privacy. Wishing you well. These acts honor what happened and protect both people from future hurt.

The internet will keep changing. New platforms will arrive. Filters will sharpen. Artificial intelligence will learn to generate images that look like anyone. Deepfakes already threaten reputations and consent. Laws will lag and then sprint. Throughout the churn, your principles can stay steady. Only share what you can stand to lose. Treat other people's bodies as you want yours treated. Speak before screens enter the room. Choose novelty that keeps you human. Protect the version of you who will read these messages in ten years and feel relief rather than dread.

You do not have to master every tool to build a satisfying digital erotic life. You need a handful of habits that you practice consistently. Ask for consent in plain words. Keep secrets out of the bedroom unless they are joyful surprises. Archive with caution. Praise the person you actually touch more than the images you scroll. Use the speed of technology to send desire ahead of you, and use the slowness of breath to receive it when you meet. If you do that steadily, your phone becomes a bridge rather than a wedge, and your screen becomes a window you can close whenever you want to return to the room where your body lives.

Chapter 14
Kink, Power, and Play: Safety, Consent, and Meaning

Power lives inside every bedroom whether people name it or not. Someone leads more often, someone receives more often, someone asks directly, someone signals with hints, someone watches for a nod before moving, someone makes the plan and someone follows; those dynamics exist in ordinary sex and in quiet affection. Kink begins when partners bring that power to the foreground, agree about it in plain words, and turn it into a creative frame for pleasure. The result can look theatrical or simple, ritualized or playful, tender or fierce. What matters is that two minds construct the scene together, care for each other's bodies, and tell meaningfully different stories than the ones handed to them by habit.

Many readers arrive here with mixed feelings. Curiosity pulls in one direction, worry in another. Some were taught that interest in bondage or impact signals damage. Others watched exaggerated media and concluded that kink must be loud, cruel, or performed for an audience. The reality inside healthy practice looks very different. Kink is a language for sensation, attention, and trust. It gives structure to exploration so that each person knows how power will move and how to stop it at any second. It adds edges that wake the nervous system, then surrounds those edges with care. When practiced well, kink reduces ambivalence because boundaries are discussed before touch begins. For many couples, that clarity is the most radical part.

Consent sits at the center of every scene. Ordinary sex often relies on context and nonverbal cues to convey yes and no. Kink asks for more than inference. Partners negotiate in advance and keep checking during play. A simple framework many communities use is Safe, Sane, Consensual. Another is Risk Aware Consensual Kink. The titles differ, the heart stays the same. You and your partner name what you want, acknowledge the risks, agree on limits, pick signals that will stop the action, and commit to aftercare. In ordinary life people sometimes treat consent as a signature on a contract. In kink consent is supervision that stays present in the room. You do not ask once and then forget. You keep listening to the body beneath the words, and you pause when anything shifts.

Negotiation sounds clinical to people who associate sex with spontaneity. In practice it can feel flirtatious and relieving. You can meet in daylight with coffee and talk about roles, activities, and edges. You can write a short scene in plain language, then read it to each other and edit. You can set a time boundary, choose a playlist, pick a few phrases that will anchor the dynamic, and decide how you want to reconnect afterward. Couples who do this once discover that details remove performance anxiety. The mind relaxes because it knows the plan and knows how to stop the plan. The body then has freedom to respond.

Signals for stopping should be short and unmistakable. The traffic light system works for many pairs: green for more, yellow for slow or change something, red for stop immediately. Some prefer a single word that never appears in ordinary arousal talk. Others agree on a hand gesture or an object dropped to the floor in case the mouth is busy. Breath play, gag use, or role play that includes resistance requires nonverbal options as primary. The promise that follows any stop matters as much as the signal itself. People need to know that a red will bring water, eye contact, calm voice, and a reset rather than pleading, disappointment, or argument. When that promise is kept repeatedly, edgy play gets safer because the nervous system learns to trust the brakes.

Newcomers often ask where to start. Think smaller than you imagine. A scene does not require rope or costumes to count as kink. It requires structure. One partner can be in charge of pace for fifteen minutes while the other commits to following guidance. One partner can be the only person allowed to speak while the other answers with touch. One partner can have permission to ask and no permission to demand. You can decide that there will be no genital contact at all, only hands on shoulders, back, and the sides of the ribs, while the receiver practices saying exactly what increases pleasure. These micro scenes rehearse consent and power without overwhelming anyone's tolerance.

Role play lives under the same rules. The goal is not acting skill. The goal is a temporary frame that helps the brain enter a different mode. Some people want to be praised explicitly for following orders. Others want to be teased for slowness or impatience inside an agreed script. Others want a teacher and student frame, or a boss and assistant frame, or a traveler and guide frame, or a celebrity and bodyguard frame, or a worshiper and altar frame that uses reverence rather than authority. What matters is that the frame fits your values and allows you to feel more alive, not less. The words you choose should be the kind you can hear the next morning without flinching. If a line poisons aftercare, retire it.

Bondage has practical and psychological facets. On the practical side you are working with posture, circulation, and nerve pathways. A single loop around wrists placed above the head changes how the chest opens, how the back arches, and how breath feels. A loop around thighs changes access and angle. A soft scarf can give a beginner the feeling of containment without the risks of complex rope. The psychology emerges from containment and focus. Many receivers report that light restraint lets them stop monitoring and surrender to sensation. Many givers report that tying or holding places their attention in the present more effectively than any mindfulness exercise. Safety requires attention to color, temperature, tingling, and numbness in the restrained limbs, frequent checks, and tools within reach to free knots quickly. Precision becomes part of care.

Impact play begins with anatomy as well. The human body has areas that tolerate sensation better than others. Muscles of the buttocks and thighs can receive rhythmic swats more comfortably than bony structures of the spine or kidneys. The rhythm matters because nerves respond to consistent patterns differently than to chaotic ones. A steady tempo relaxes many bodies even when the sensations are strong, while erratic hits can trigger vigilance and anxiety. Communication in the middle is more important than in many other practices. The receiver can say faster, slower, softer, higher, lower, stay, change to the other side, pause for breath. The giver matches that input and watches the body more than the face, because many receivers drift into altered attention and speak less. If the skin tears or bruises appear where they were not wanted, aftercare includes cleaning, ointment, and time. If marks are welcome, you can photograph them later with the same consent rules you use for any intimate images. Many couples discover that impact play becomes tender precisely because it requires those discussions.

Power exchange does not depend on pain. Many scenes omit it entirely. A dominant partner can control pace and language while giving only gentle touch. A submissive partner can ask permission for each movement and receive praise for attention.

A top can lead a meditation, direct breath, and hold the receiver's jaw while speaking slowly. A bottom can kneel on soft pillows and close their eyes while committing to stillness. These quieter scenes are not a lesser form. For many nervous systems they are the entry point because they keep arousal inside safety.

Breath and voice turn out to be more powerful than most beginners expect. When the person in the lead slows their own breathing, counts the receiver's inhale out loud, and asks them to match a longer exhale, sensations change immediately. Tone of voice can increase intensity faster than speed of touch. A low, steady tone with deliberate pauses communicates that the person in charge is paying attention, which allows the receiver to let go. The reverse is true when tone tightens or becomes clipped. Many misses in kink scenes come from mismatched nervous systems. The leader sprints. The follower tries to keep up. The fix is physiological. Slow the leader until the follower's breath meets it. Then build together.

Aftercare is not optional theater. It is the recovery phase of a shared exertion. The body, after arousal peaks or after intense emotion, needs help descending. A blanket, a glass of water, a snack, a warm cloth for skin, eye contact, and a few sentences about what worked, all of this tells the nervous system that the story ended well. After role play that included harsh words, aftercare may need explicit apology inside the frame. Thank you for trusting me. I know those words do not belong to us outside this scene. Are you comfortable. Do you want silence, humor, or praise. Many receivers drop into a calm state after intense scenes and feel sleepy or tender for an hour. Others feel energized and chatty. Others feel emotional, even tearful. Plan for these states rather than being surprised by them. The debrief belongs a little later, when both of you can think clearly. Then you can talk about what you would adjust next time and praise what you want repeated.

People with trauma histories can enjoy kink, provided that consent is substantial and pacing is slow. Some survivors find that power exchange gives back control. Others discover that certain words or positions trigger flashbacks. The only rule is to stay inside tolerance. You can treat kink as graded exposure, starting with tiny doses that remain gentle and predictable. You can use self-tying or self-directed scenes as practice before inviting a partner in. You can reclaim words that once hurt you by placing them inside a script where you hold authority. Or you can ban those words forever and still have a rich erotic life. Nothing in this chapter requires reenactment of harm. The point is to widen choices and increase agency, not to reproduce old pain.

Neurodivergent partners often flourish in kink spaces because rules are explicit. A written plan calms an autistic mind that dislikes ambiguity. Clear hand signals keep an ADHD mind oriented when sensation pulls attention away from language. Sensory preferences can be honored without apology. Low light, consistent rhythm, limited eye contact during peak sensation, and predictable sequence reduce overload. The leader can narrate transitions. The follower can hold a card with stop signals if speech goes offline. Far from killing passion, these supports make intensity possible.

Disability does not disqualify anyone from power exchange. Chairs can become thrones. Pillows can turn beds into supportive platforms. Rope that once held wrists can be tied loosely around thighs to cue stillness without preventing it. A cane can become a symbol of authority rather than a reminder of loss. People with chronic pain can do short scenes with extended aftercare. People with limited grip strength can use gloves or toys that transfer effort to larger muscles. Communication about fatigue and flare patterns matters more than costumes ever will. Many disabled readers report that kink finally gave them ways to be desired as they are, rather than as a fantasy of independence.

Risk management is part of erotic care, and it looks practical. Keep first aid supplies nearby. Learn about circulation and nerve compression. Use safety shears for rope. Avoid alcohol when you plan intense scenes. Treat toys as you would kitchen tools, with cleaning protocols that do not rely on guesswork. In anal play, choose lube that lasts and toys with flared bases. In any practice with potential for skin breakage, discuss safer sex realistically. Kink communities sometimes talk about safety with reverence because that talk saves scenes from mishap and reputations from harm. Safe practice makes room for pleasure.

Meaning travels through kink in ways that often surprise people. Submission can feel like rest when life requires constant leadership. Dominance can feel like service when it concentrates attention on a partner's state. Bondage can feel like relief when the mind never stops planning. Impact can feel like clarity when numbness has been the background for months. Role play can feel like self-repair when praise inside a script rewrites sentences that once shamed you. None of this collapses into a single explanation. It simply illustrates that erotic frames talk to the parts of us that crave order, intensity, permission, or surrender. Healthy kink tells those parts that they can eat without eating the rest of the self.

Couples who want to explore together can begin with a conversation that names a shared curiosity. One person might say that watchfulness during sex makes it hard to feel, and that they want to try surrendering decisions for a short time. The other might say that they crave direct praise and want to be told exactly what to do with their hands and mouth. From there a small plan emerges. Tonight we will do twenty minutes. You will kneel on a folded blanket by the bed and keep your eyes closed. I will touch your shoulders and speak in a low voice.

There will be no penetration. Your job is to breathe slowly and tell me what happens in your body. My job is to stay steady and watch you carefully. Afterward we will drink water and lie still. We will talk later. That level of detail sounds simple and functions as a scaffold strong enough to hold trust.

For readers who want to explore communities, the same consent rules apply at scale. Look for events that post clear codes of conduct, welcome newcomers, emphasize education, and enforce boundaries. Observe before you engage. Notice how people speak to staff and to each other. Watch how consent is obtained, how scenes stop, and how aftercare appears. Communities that treat volunteers well tend to treat attendees well. If the culture prizes invincibility, leave. If it prizes care, you are more likely to learn in safety.

Long distance partners can integrate power exchange through words and schedules. A morning message can set a tone for the day and a night message can close the frame. A shared document can carry rules that both agree serve connection rather than control, such as when the follower will take breaks for water or stretches, or when the leader will send praise. App-connected toys can be used in windows that respect time zones and work life. Video scenes require the same consent and aftercare as in-person scenes. The added work is narrating more, since touch cannot carry the meaning.

Religion and ethics do not sit outside kink. They sit inside it. People of faith can build scenes that honor their values, framing power as stewardship and care rather than domination for its own sake. They can retire words that conflict with conscience and choose others that carry reverence. Couples can include prayer or gratitude in aftercare. Communities can insist on dignity and inclusion so that kink culture does not reproduce the very harms many of its participants came to escape. Ethics kept close to the body feel less like rules and more like a promise: we will not hurt each other's humanity in the name of pleasure.

Shame often recedes when people tell the truth to someone safe. You can say out loud that you want to be tied and touched gently until you cry, and that the crying would be relief. You can say that you want to order someone to hold still and then praise them for the skill of stillness. You can say that you want to be called beautiful while you kneel. You can say that you want to sprawl and be looked at and be told you are wanted in words you never received. The surface details vary. The structure remains the same. Two people bring hunger to a table and feed each other carefully.

Misses will happen. A knot will pinch. A line will land wrong. A mark will be darker than expected. Repair follows the same steps as in any intimacy. Stop. Care for the body. Care for the emotions. Debrief later. Decide what to change. Keep or retire the practice. The reputation that kink has for drama usually rests on scenes where consent was assumed rather than negotiated. When negotiation is ordinary, repair becomes ordinary too, and the relationship stays light enough for play.

A few practical scripts close the gap between reading and doing. If you want to lead, you can say, I want to set a scene where I control pace for twenty minutes. There will be no penetration. Your job is to breathe and tell me if anything changes. Are you willing. If you want to follow, you can say, I want to give you control for a short time, and I want to know exactly how we will stop. Can we use red to stop and promise to pause for water and holding. If you want impact play, you can say, I am curious about five minutes of spanking on my thighs and buttocks. Please start soft and stay steady. I will say yellow if I need less and green if I want more. If you want role play, you can say, I want to be praised while I follow instructions. Avoid insults.

Use my name. End by telling me that you are proud of me. These sentences remove guesswork, which reduces fear.

For those who worry that kink will replace tenderness, consider this: tenderness grows in rooms where people feel seen. When you ask for power exchange and receive it with care, you are not stepping away from love. You are stepping toward a version of it that speaks to nerves and breath in ways conventional sex never did for you. Many couples report that ordinary touch becomes sweeter after structured scenes because the residue of unspoken roles is gone. They have played at power honestly. The rest of life can be more equal again.

A final picture may help. Imagine a couple on a Wednesday night. The dishwasher hums. A lamp warms the corner of the room. They have a plan written in a few lines on a card. The leader will sit on the edge of the bed and hold the follower's jaw with one hand while the other rests on the follower's chest to feel breath. There will be simple commands. Open your eyes. Close them. Inhale through your nose. Hold. Exhale. Good. The follower will keep their hands on their thighs and receive touch without reaching. There will be no sex during the scene. A timer will ring at fifteen minutes. Afterward they will drink water and lie with the follower's head on the leader's shoulder. Later that week they will talk about what worked and what changed. Nothing flashy occurred. Everything important did. Attention, power, care, and consent braided themselves into a memory that tells both bodies the same story: this is a safe place to feel.

Kink is not required for a healthy erotic life, yet for many it becomes a reliable path to desire because it organizes attention and gives permission. When practiced with respect, it deepens trust rather than risking it, expands vocabulary rather than shrinking it, and turns sex into a craft two people work on together. The point is not to collect costumes or scenes. The point is to grow the capacity to play with intensity and then return each other gently to the rest of life. If you keep that aim in view, power becomes a tool you share rather than a weight you drag, and pleasure becomes easier to find inside the bodies and the values you already have.

Chapter 15
Queer, Trans, and Nonconforming Sexualities

Sex education in many places was written for a narrow room. Straight couples filled the examples. Cisgender bodies filled the diagrams. Anyone who did not fit that frame learned by inference, by rumor, by trial, and often by hiding. This chapter widens the room on purpose. Queer, trans, nonbinary, intersex, asexual, aromantic, kinky, polyamorous, and otherwise nonconforming readers deserve language that treats their experiences as ordinary parts of human sexuality. Partners who identify as straight and cisgender benefit too, because the same clarity, consent, anatomy knowledge, and respect that support queer and trans pleasure also make heterosexual sex better.

Identity begins as a felt truth and then becomes a life. Orientation describes the patterns of who you are drawn to emotionally, romantically, and sexually. Gender describes how your sense of self relates to the social categories of woman, man, both, neither, or something more fluid. Bodies have parts. Identities have meaning. Attraction has direction. Relationships have structure. Many adults were told that these four domains collapse into one bundle that never changes. Real lives refuse that bundle. A lesbian woman can be nonbinary. A bisexual man can be monogamous for twenty years. A trans woman can love women. An asexual person can have a rich sensual life. A gay man can be kinky and also domestic and tender. Precision helps because precision allows pleasure to follow what is true rather than what is assumed.

History matters because scripts carry weight. Most queer and trans people learned early to scan rooms for danger. That vigilance kept them safe and also became a habit that sometimes enters bed. When someone checks the door and the window twice before a kiss, the nervous system is doing its job. When a partner asks for slower pace and more words before touch, the nervous system is asking for a chance to switch from protection to connection. Sex that honors this history feels different. It begins with consent that is specific. It continues with language that names bodies as they are and wishes as they are. It ends with aftercare that includes appreciation for honesty and courage, because those qualities are part of the arousal context for many queer and trans people.

Language about bodies should serve the person who lives in the body. Default labels often fail here. Some trans women prefer the word vagina for their neovagina after vaginoplasty, while others prefer surgical vagina or simply vagina without qualifiers. Some trans men call their genitals a front hole or a vagina, and some prefer cock for a hormonally enlarged clitoris. Nonbinary people choose terms that fit their sense of self and change them over time. Partners can ask which words land well and then use them consistently. This is not politeness for its own sake. The right word removes friction in the mind and allows attention to return to sensation.

Anatomy and hormones shape pleasure in ways that deserve practical notes. Testosterone often increases genital sensitivity, enlarges the clitoris, and changes lubrication patterns. Estrogen can reduce spontaneous erections over time and increase breast sensitivity. Puberty blockers used in adolescence alter the timing of puberty, which can influence adult arousal patterns and the meaning of certain touches. Surgical procedures add variables. A neovagina requires dilation and lubrication practices that vary by technique. Phalloplasty and metoidioplasty change erectile tissue and nerve distribution, which shifts preferred angles and pressures. Top surgery changes how chest sensation travels through the nervous system. None of these changes erase sexuality. They simply alter the map. Couples who treat each transition as an opportunity to relearn rather than as a loss tend to find stable routes back to pleasure.

Consent scripts make queer and trans sex safer and hotter at the same time. Many readers carry old experiences with misgendering, fetishization, or coerced disclosure. A partner who begins with questions that respect boundaries builds trust quickly. You can ask which parts want touch today and which parts want to be left alone. You can ask which words for your partner's body feel affirming. You can ask whether there are topics or kinks that should wait for another time. Then you can offer your own map with the same precision. Clarity lowers vigilance. Lower vigilance makes room for arousal.

Arousal nonconcordance can be pronounced in contexts where identity is on the line. A body can respond to stimulation while the mind hesitates because language is wrong or because the dynamic feels off. In those moments the wise choice is to slow down, name the mismatch, and adjust. A sentence such as my body is responding and I am still catching up emotionally keeps both people inside one story. When partners normalize this check-in, sex remains connected even when the pace changes.

Queer sex is sometimes described as a set of acts between genitals. The richer description sees it as a set of skills between minds. Negotiation of roles, consent to power exchange, decisions about barriers, agreements about disclosure, and respect for chosen family are as central to queer erotic life as any technique. Straight readers who adopt these skills discover that sex becomes easier because everyone knows the plan. Queer readers do not need permission to claim this tradition. They built it.

Safety in public spaces affects libido at home. A person who is misgendered at work, questioned in bathrooms, stared at while holding hands, or threatened on transit often arrives at night with a nervous system that is still active. Partners who understand this reality do not take the distance personally. They change the conditions. They slow the evening, protect privacy, add time for warm up, and take turns carrying the mental load of vigilance in daily life so that both people can rest sometimes. Many couples discover that a fair division of political and logistical labor is an aphrodisiac.

Asexual and aromantic experiences need direct inclusion. Some people rarely or never feel sexual attraction. Some people rarely or never feel romantic attraction. Some feel both in limited ways or under specific conditions. None of these profiles disqualify someone from intimacy. Many ace and aro folks enjoy touch, sensuality, partnership, co-parenting, or kink within carefully negotiated parameters. The key is transparency early and often. A partner who hears I enjoy sensual closeness and do not want genital sex can decide whether that structure fits their life. When consent includes honest limits, relationships remain respectful even when desires differ.

Bisexual and pansexual readers carry unique strain in cultures that prefer tidy categories. Some partners assume that bi people are more likely to cheat. Some communities ask bi people to choose a side. The nervous system hears those pressures and braces. Breadth of attraction does not translate to breadth of betrayal. What predicts trust is the same for everyone. People who keep agreements and repair misses remain trustworthy. People who hide and excuse remain risky. Naming this truth clearly removes a layer of stigma that harms sex for no benefit.

Monogamy and nonmonogamy need equal respect. Queer communities invented many of the modern tools for ethical nonmonogamy, and they also contain couples who choose exclusivity for reasons that suit them. The structure matters less than the clarity of agreements. Who knows about whom. What kind of contact is in bounds. How will safer sex be handled. What aftercare do partners expect after outside encounters. How will jealousy be named and metabolized. When those questions are answered in daylight, erotic life has room to breathe. When they are ignored, people end up policing each other instead of building intimacy.

Pleasure techniques deserve detail because many queer and trans readers were handed silence. For vulva owners, external stimulation remains the most reliable route to orgasm across orientations and genders. Pressure and rhythm that focus on the clitoral hood and labia work for many. For penis owners, consistent strokes that include the frenulum and glans, paired with attention to breathing and pelvic floor relaxation, remain effective even when hormones or surgery alter blood flow. Anal pleasure can be rich for people of all genders, provided that preparation, lubrication, patience, and communication stay central. Trans women who tuck daily may benefit from gentle external massage before more focused touch to ease tension. Trans men on testosterone may prefer firmer pressure or different angles as the clitoris enlarges. Nonbinary people may enjoy alternating between names and techniques that affirm different facets of self within one scene. Precision is the point. Your partner's body today deserves a map that was written today.

Pain and dysphoria require special care. Dysphoria can spike when attention lands on a body part that conflicts with identity. You can mitigate this with lighting, clothing, positions, and language that keep attention on areas that feel congruent. A trans woman who dislikes direct genital focus may want hands on thighs, hips, breasts, and face, with orgasm arriving through thigh squeezing or toy use rather than through penile stimulation. A trans man who prefers to avoid the word vagina may enjoy touch described as cock play and positions that frame his genitals as a cock, with toys that match that frame. When pain appears, especially after surgery or with hormonal shifts, the solution is clinical care plus adjustments to technique. No one earns gender or orientation by enduring discomfort.

Disclosure and privacy are part of consent. Partners have a right to safety. People have a right to choose when and how to share identity or history. Dating while trans or nonbinary often involves a discussion about timing. Some disclose in profiles to protect themselves from violence and to filter for partners who are ready. Others disclose in messages before meeting. Others disclose in person once safety is clear. There is no single correct order. The rule that never changes is this: no one is entitled to anyone's body. Consent can be revoked at any point without reason. People who respond to disclosure with curiosity and care create rooms where sex can happen. People who respond with fetishizing questions or pressure do not.

Healthcare access remains a core sexual issue for queer and trans communities. Primary care providers who ask about partners without assuming gender help patients relax. Gynecologists who offer trauma informed exams and who know how to examine a neovagina without causing harm preserve function. Urologists who understand the sexual side effects of testosterone blockers treat trans women as whole people. Mental health clinicians who can speak about identity without turning every concern into identity reduce isolation. Readers can interview providers and leave those who cannot meet this standard. Your body and your identity deserve competence and respect at the same time.

Religion and culture influence queer and trans erotic life in specific ways. Some readers hold faith traditions that told them to disappear. Others hold communities that celebrate them. Many live between those poles. Health grows where values about fidelity, honesty, care for the vulnerable, and dignity for all bodies remain, while rules that punish desire or erase identities fall away. A couple can observe sabbath and still plan sensual time. A person can belong to a church and still require their pastor to use correct pronouns. A family can honor ancestors and still celebrate a child's new name. Alignment between values and daily life reduces shame. Reduced shame increases desire.

Chosen family supports sex directly because it supports the person. Friends who use correct names and pronouns, who respect partners, who show up during illness and transition, become part of the context that allows erotic life to flourish. Many queer couples thrive because the relationship is held by a web of care that distributes stress and celebrates milestones. Straight readers can build similar webs. Community keeps desire from being crushed by logistics.

Porn and erotica deserve a careful look because representation changes arousal context. Queer and trans viewers often look for material that mirrors their bodies and desires without humiliation or violence. When they find it, arousal rises more easily because the mind does not have to fight the images. When they cannot find it, imagination carries more weight. Couples can create their own erotic scripts, write scenes that fit their ethics, and read them aloud. Audio erotica that names bodies accurately can support trans and nonbinary arousal when visuals in mainstream porn feel dissonant.

Youth deserve specific guidance. Queer and trans teens live under higher surveillance in many places and under higher risk of harm. Adults who care can teach consent, safer sex, and pleasure in ways that reflect the identities in the room. Accurate condom and dental dam use should be taught for oral and anal sex. Lubricant should be normalized for all kinds of sex. Pronouns should be respected in classrooms and clinics. Names should be honored. Teens who learn that their identities are valid are more likely to seek care and less likely to be exploited.

Aging inside queer and trans communities brings changes worth naming. Hormone regimens shift. Surgeries need ongoing care. Partners die and chosen family becomes crucial. Desire often slows and deepens. Many older queer adults report relief at the reduction of social scrutiny, which allows them to savor sex without the pressure to represent anyone. Medical systems must catch up by asking about partners, by screening appropriately regardless of anatomy, and by including sexual health questions in routine care. Pleasure belongs to elders as much as to youth.

Practical scripts help partners move from ideals to actions. Before a first sexual encounter you can say I want to check language for our bodies so that we both feel good. I like these words for me. Which words do you want. Before initiating you can say I am feeling close and want to touch your chest and your hips. Do you want that tonight. During touch you can say tell me if there is any shift in comfort, and I will adjust or stop. Afterward you can say I loved the way you guided my hand and I want to try that rhythm again. These sentences protect dignity while feeding arousal.

Shame fades in rooms where people tell the truth and receive respect. A trans man can say that he wants to be called handsome and wanted and that he prefers touch that treats his genitals as a cock. A nonbinary person can say that they want to be seen outside of categories and that their arousal grows when a partner narrates what is beautiful about their shape and voice.

A lesbian couple can say that they want to retire scripts that center penetration and let external stimulation count as complete. A gay couple can say that they want to de-emphasize performance and build scenes that honor rest as much as intensity. Each declaration clears a path for pleasure.

Conflict shows up here like anywhere else. Partners will misstep with pronouns. Old habits will appear in bed. Jealousy will rise. Avoidance will return after a painful night. Repair works the same way. Name the harm without theatrics. Apologize without self-defense. Ask for what would restore trust. Offer a concrete change. Set a review date. Desire returns near that kind of accountability because the nervous system learns that safety is not a wish. It is a practice.

The center of the chapter is simple. Queer, trans, and nonconforming sexualities do not require special permission to be healthy. They require accurate maps, supportive community, competent care, and partners who listen. Bodies that have been policed need contexts that feel free. Identities that have been doubted need daily affirmation. Relationships that have been told they are impossible need ordinary logistics, shopping lists, calendars, and inside jokes. When those supports exist, arousal behaves like arousal in any human. It rises when conditions are right, it pauses when conditions are wrong, and it returns when people create better conditions together.

If you are reading as a queer or trans person, consider pausing to list what helps your body arrive. Include words, settings, clothing, times of day, safety signals, and aftercare that works. Then share that list with someone you trust or keep it as your own guide. If you are reading as a straight, cis partner who wants to love well, consider listing what you do not know yet and committing to learn without asking your partner to carry all the teaching. If you are reading as a parent or teacher or clinician, consider which habit you can change this week that will make one queer or trans person safer. Each action increases the zone where pleasure can happen.

Sexual health belongs to everyone in this room. Health here means consent that is real, bodies that are named correctly, protection that reflects actual practices, repair that respects dignity, and joy that fits the people present. The broader culture will keep changing. Laws will move. Representation will rise and fall. Inside those shifts, your bedroom and your body can remain places where truth and kindness lead. When they do, sex becomes less about passing for normal and more about living what is honest, connected, and deeply yours.

Chapter 16
Monogamy, Nonmonogamy:
How to Design the Relationship
You Actually Want

Most of us inherited one default model of love. Find one person, fall for each other, blend sex with affection, promise exclusivity, and keep the promise forever. Many people thrive inside that frame when they treat it as a living agreement rather than as a story that runs itself. Others discover they want something different. The goal of this chapter is not to sell one structure over another. The goal is to teach design. When you know how to name values, write agreements, handle jealousy, protect health, and repair trust, you can build monogamy that stays alive or consensual nonmonogamy that stays kind.

Begin with the foundation that holds any structure together. Tell the truth about what you want, and give your partner the right to want something else. People try to keep love by hiding appetite or hiding limits. Secrets feel safer at the start and cost more later. A couple that admits they want strict exclusivity has the same dignity as a couple that admits they want a wider field. What matters is consent that is informed, ongoing, and practical.

Monogamy works best when it is explicit. Many couples pledge fidelity without defining it. Trouble arrives in the gap between assumptions. You can bring the edges into daylight. Describe which behaviors count as sexual or romantic contact outside the relationship. Name whether flirting at a party feels fun or threatening. Decide whether texting with an ex is welcome or whether that contact needs a boundary. Agree on how to handle attractions that surprise you. Decide what you both want from privacy and what you both want from transparency. Say out loud how each of you will ask for help if desire dips or if someone else's attention wakes something up. This is not overkill. This is how you stop guessing and start building.

Exclusivity also benefits from nutrition. Relationships that only police the perimeter grow brittle. Feed the inside with steady care. Schedule intimacy windows that match your bodies. Keep a habit of repair after misses. Protect sleep. Share labor fairly so that nobody arrives in bed with a running to-do list while the other arrives with free attention. Design novelty that does not threaten the bond. A new room. A new time of day. A different sequence. A negotiated fantasy that belongs only to you two. Many couples who feared boredom discover that boredom is a sign of underfeeding, not a verdict on love.

Consensual nonmonogamy comes in many shapes. Some couples keep sex outside the bond casual and private from the rest of life. Some create friendships that include sex. Some invite a third person into their shared home. Some open briefly during travel. Some practice swinging where experiences happen together. Some build polyamorous networks where multiple loving relationships are named and sustained. Labels simplify conversations, yet they never replace the work of precise agreements. Your version must fit your nervous systems, your schedules, your health needs, your community, and your values.

Openings begin well when they begin slowly. Curiosity sounds different from urgency. Curiosity asks what problem you hope opening will solve and whether that problem has solutions inside the relationship. Curiosity asks what excites you and what scares you. Curiosity asks how much time and energy you actually have for additional relationships. Urgency skips the questions and crashes the calendar. Urgency often hides resentment or avoidance. If you are asking to open because you hope to escape a painful dynamic at home, you are likely to carry the pain into the next room. Repair first, then open, or agree that you will address both simultaneously with clear checkpoints so that the primary bond does not become an afterthought.

Agreements protect everyone only when they are practical. Choose a cadence for testing and stick to it. Decide which barriers you will use for which activities with outside partners. Name who will be told about whom and when, including friends and family. Decide how you want to handle digital traces such as messages and photos. Plan how you will disclose your structure to new people and what you will do if someone reacts with pressure or confusion. Decide where first meetings will happen and how you will get home. Name how you will manage contraception if pregnancy is possible for anyone involved. Choose language for aftercare following dates that honors the primary relationship without treating other people as disposable.

Time is love's currency. Opening a relationship spends time by definition. Couples who do this well budget deliberately. If you plan one date with someone new, plan one date with each other. If you devote a weekend away to another relationship, schedule an equal weekend for the two of you as soon as possible. If you anticipate a season of high novelty with someone else, triple your check-ins with your primary partner. Nothing erodes security faster than uncertainty about where resources will go. You can keep the ledger human and still keep it precise.

Jealousy is not a failure of character. It is an emotion that carries information. Jealousy often hides a request. The request may be for reassurance that you are wanted. The request may be for predictability about time. The request may be for respect around introductions. The request may be for temporary limits while a particular outside connection feels destabilizing. Couples who name the request find a path. Couples who moralize the feeling get stuck arguing about whether jealousy should exist. It exists. Treat it like weather. You bring umbrellas, you change plans when needed, and you do not insult the rain.

Compersion is a word many people use to describe the pleasure of watching a partner enjoy someone else. Do not force it. For some nervous systems it emerges naturally when security is high and when partners are careful about time, care, and disclosure. For others it never appears, and that does not make them small. The opposite of compersion is not cruelty. The opposite is neutrality. If you feel neutral about your partner's outside connection and remain loving toward your partner, you are doing the work. Pressuring yourself toward joy will make you brittle. Aim for steadiness and keep practicing the behaviors that keep steadiness possible.

New relationship energy is real. Novelty pours dopamine and norepinephrine into attention. Texts seem bright. Plans seem easy. Flaws seem charming. People often mistake this state for a verdict on old love. It is a verdict on novelty, not on worth. Couples that survive NRE keep rituals in place. Good morning and good night still belong to the home relationship unless you have agreed differently. Important news still comes home first. Birthdays and anniversaries remain protected. If you are the person caught in the glow, invite your partner to tell you where the glow is burning the house and change behavior fast. You can enjoy excitement without disrespecting the base you stand on.

Disclosure deserves detail. Some people want a complete debrief after every outside date. Some want broad strokes. Others only want to know what affects health or schedule. Find a level that prevents secrets from growing while also protecting each person's autonomy. If your partner needs fewer details, restrain the impulse to soothe your anxiety by over sharing. If your partner needs more details, restrain the impulse to hide because you fear their feelings. Choose the smallest honest version that keeps both of you steady, then adjust with experience.

Metamours are partners of your partner. They are not your enemies. Healthy networks treat each other as people with needs, not as obstacles or trophies. Your metamour does not owe you intimacy. They do owe you basic respect and adherence to the agreements that keep everyone safe. Some networks flourish with friendly contact among metamours. Others keep polite distance. Conflict often dissolves when everyone remembers that the shared aim is each person's thriving, not victory in a rivalry that no one consented to.

Children and family life can coexist with open structures, provided that adults plan carefully. Kids need stability, privacy, and honest answers at developmentally appropriate levels. They do not need to meet every person their parents date. They do not need to hear adult details. They do need to know who will pick them up from school and who will be at the dinner table. If a long-term partner becomes part of family life, introduce gradually and keep the child's routines intact. Many families choose to say that they have close friends who are important. As children age, language can widen if the adults prefer. The principle remains the same. Protect the child's sense of safety and dignity.

Religious and cultural values matter here as much as anywhere else. Some readers hold beliefs that root sexual exclusivity in covenant. Others hold beliefs that root ethics in care and consent more than in structure. You can align a relationship with your values without insisting that other structures are inferior. If you choose exclusivity, you can set it in language that honors desire rather than subduing it. If you choose openness, you can set it in language that honors commitment rather than eroding it. Values that center honesty, care for the vulnerable, and responsibility for consequences will protect any structure you choose.

Health practices cannot be optional in open networks. Testing has to become a routine, not a reaction. Many people choose quarterly screening when they have outside partners or add a test after any new connection that includes fluid exchange. Condoms, internal condoms, dental dams, and gloves belong in nightstands and travel kits. Lubricant reduces microtears and lowers risk. Apps that store results can simplify disclosure, and written agreements about who informs whom after an exposure prevent panic on hard days. Treat these steps as part of intimacy rather than as intrusions. Protecting bodies is one way lovers say I care about your future.

Digital boundaries deserve the same care as physical boundaries. Decide whether phones are open books or private devices. Decide whether location sharing reduces fear or increases surveillance. Decide what happens to photos if a connection ends. Decide how often you will be reachable while on outside dates and what messages count as urgent. Decide which details belong in group chats and which belong in direct conversations only. These are not technicalities. These decisions prevent ruptures that have little to do with sex and everything to do with attention and respect.

Breaks and closures are part of honest design. There will be seasons when exclusivity grows again because a crisis needs all available energy. There will be seasons when you pause outside contact because jealousy flares and requires repair. There will be seasons when a particular connection ends because the fit was wrong or because someone was careless with agreements.

Closures go better when you practice care. Inform people directly and promptly. Do not ghost. Return belongings. Delete private media as promised. Speak about former partners kindly to anyone who was not part of the connection. You are building a reputation that will follow you into the next season.

Breach of agreement is different from exploration that stays within consent. A breach needs repair that is specific and sustained. The person who broke the agreement must take responsibility without minimizing impact. The person who was hurt must be allowed to feel angry, sad, or numb without being pressed to forgive quickly. Together you set a period where transparency increases. Together you choose whether you need a pause on outside contact. Together you schedule extra time for connection and for clinical care if trauma symptoms appear. Together you set a review date to decide whether trust is rebuilding. Couples that rush this process repeat it. Couples that slow down and do each step discover whether the relationship can hold.

Monogamy deserves a section on renewal because many readers want exclusivity and worry that it will dim. You can renew by building a small ritual for desire. Pick a weekly window that belongs to sex even if sex becomes a massage or a shower together that ends with kisses and sleep. Trade initiation for a month so that both of you develop the muscles that keep erotic energy circulating. Share fantasies at the level of theme and translate one into action each quarter. Create a habit of sending one message a week that names something you want to do with the person you already love. Speak appreciation out loud. Desire feeds on being wanted by a specific someone who knows you.

Polyamory deserves a section on sustainability because many readers imagine abundance without counting costs. Multiple relationships require time, travel, money, and emotional labor. People who thrive create calendars that show commitments at a glance and leave buffers for rest. They check in with themselves weekly about capacity and say no when overflow threatens everyone's health. They learn to tolerate the discomfort of missing moments so that they can savor the moments they actually live. Abundance is not the number of people who could say yes. Abundance is the amount of presence you can bring to the people you have chosen.

A note for readers who prefer relationship anarchy or other models that discard hierarchy entirely. You can live without ranking partners while still practicing reliability. The skills remain the same. Communicate intentions clearly. Keep boundaries you name. Give aftercare to people you touch. Inform partners about health status. Do not make promises you cannot keep. When a conflict of needs arises, name it early and negotiate in good faith rather than disappearing. Freedom without reliability leaves a wake of confusion that eventually returns to your own door.

Scripts help when you feel brave and awkward at the same time. To open a conversation about exclusivity you can say I love us and want to keep us strong. Let us write down what monogamy means for us so that we do not assume and then stumble. To raise the idea of opening you can say curiosity is here for me, and I want to explore together without rushing. My hope is more aliveness and more honesty. My fear is distance. Can we start with a month of talking and then one small experiment with a review date. To handle jealousy you can say the feeling landed today and I need reassurance about time and wanting. Please tell me our next two dates and one thing you are eager to do with me. To set health terms with a new partner you can say I use barriers for all genital contact and I test quarterly. I will inform you and my other partners if anything changes. Are you willing to match this practice.

Therapy helps many couples design well. A therapist who understands sexual diversity can slow the conversation when urgency appears, translate values into agreements, and hold both sides steady when early attempts feel clumsy. Coaching from educators who specialize in open structures can supplement therapy by adding scripts, calendars, and health practices that save you from learning every lesson the hard way. If a clinician tells you your interest in openness proves immaturity, find a clinician who can hold nuance. If a clinician tells you your interest in exclusivity proves insecurity, find a clinician who respects choice. Good helpers protect consent, dignity, and health, not a single ideology.

Measure success with the right yardsticks. A healthy monogamous relationship is not one that never faces temptation. It is one that handles desire transparently and keeps feeding the bond. A healthy open relationship is not one that never feels jealous. It is one that honors feelings without letting them run the ship and keeps everyone safer than they would be alone. In both structures, kindness to the people you touch is nonnegotiable. If your choices require someone else to feel small or kept in the dark, your design needs new plans.

End with a picture of craft. Two people sit at a kitchen table with calendars, tea, and the habit of listening. They review the last month. They name what worked. They admit what hurt. They adjust a few boundaries and schedule two different kinds of dates, one playful and one tender. They confirm health plans and travel plans. They praise what they want repeated. They leave the table with a map that both can carry. Nothing magical happened. They did the work. That is how love in any structure keeps its shape.

You are allowed to choose the relationship you want. You are allowed to change your mind. You are allowed to insist on safety. You are allowed to ask for aliveness. When you design with care, sex becomes easier to trust, because it happens inside agreements that fit the two of you rather than inside a template that never met your bodies.

Chapter 17
Building a Personal Sexual Wellbeing Plan

A satisfying sexual life rarely grows on its own for years without attention. Early chemistry can feel effortless and decisive; routines, stress, illness, caregiving, grief, medications, and changing identities then arrive and the old autopilot stops working. A personal plan brings structure to a part of life that deserves care. The aim here is not to create homework that drags on desire. The aim is to design conditions that make pleasure easier to reach, safety easier to protect, and intimacy easier to sustain. Think of this chapter as a workshop you complete with a pen in hand. The result is a living document that you revise when seasons change.

Begin with a vision that fits your values. People try to fix technique while skipping purpose. Write a short paragraph that names the qualities you want in this part of your life. Some readers choose steady and connected, others choose exploratory and playful, others choose unrushed and affectionate. Then add a sentence about the kind of person you want to be during sex: honest, kind, responsive, reliable, curious. This paragraph is the compass. When choices arrive, you compare them with the compass and decide whether they move you toward or away from your stated direction.

Translate vision into principles that you can act on. Consent must be real and easy to communicate. Health practices must be practical. Privacy must protect the people involved. Repair must be routine. Pleasure must be legitimate for every participant. Write those words in your own language and keep them visible. A plan that keeps principles on the first page tends to survive hard weeks because you are less likely to improvise from anxiety.

Context mapping comes next because arousal depends on where the body lives. The accelerator responds to cues of safety, closeness, time, novelty, praise, warmth, and privacy. The brake responds to cues of stress, resentment, pain, shame, distraction, fear, and obligation. Sketch your week in plain detail. Note work intensity, commuting time, childcare blocks, exercise windows, social demands, menstrual cycle patterns if relevant, and the hours when you feel mentally available. Patterns usually appear fast. Evenings may be noisy and thin on patience. Mornings may hold more cooperation from the nervous system. Weekends may carry recovery rather than romance unless protected. Design the when of sex to suit the real day you live. People who stop fighting their circadian and social context often discover that "low desire" was a context problem with a straightforward fix.

Space carries weight. Bedrooms send messages through light, temperature, sound, clutter, fabrics, and smells. Decide what you want the room to say before you enter as a lover. A lamp that can dim, a drawer with lube and a clean towel, music that matches your pace, a lock that actually locks, bedding that does not itch, these details lower vigilance. Remove devices when you can. If phones must stay nearby for caregiving or work, turn off previews on the lock screen and place the devices outside of direct sight so that attention remains with the person or with your own body.

Body literacy belongs in every plan. Many adults never learned basic anatomy in language that dignifies pleasure. If you own a vulva, map the labia, the clitoral hood, the glans, the shaft, the crura that extend along the pelvis, the vestibule, the urethral opening, the entrance of the vagina, and the perineum.

Note how indirect touch often prepares direct touch to feel good. If you own a penis, map the shaft, the glans, the coronal ridge, the frenulum, the base, the perineum, and the pelvic floor muscles that tense and release during arousal and orgasm. If you enjoy anal play, include the external sphincter, the internal sphincter, the rectal ampulla, and the prostate when present. Write down the pressures, angles, and rhythms that usually help. Include positions that protect comfort: side lying for low back concerns, receiver on top for depth control, pillows that change angle for cervical sensitivity. A good map is not a romance novel. It is engineering language that saves nights from guesswork.

Create your personal yeses and no-for-nows. People carry inherited scripts that narrow choices without serving health. You can set your own menu. Count external stimulation as complete sex, not as a preface. Count mutual masturbation with praise and eye contact as a valid date, not as a fallback. Count a long kiss with no other goal as a success on weeks when energy is scarce. Set aside acts that irritate tissue or spike dysphoria until care is in place. Tell the truth about anal play: preparation, patience, lubrication, and communication are required; toys must have flared bases; start smaller than you think you need; stop at the first sharp sensation; breathe.

Name your brakes clearly and design around them. Common brakes include unfinished fights, unequal household labor, sensory overload, hormonal shifts, pelvic pain, erection unpredictability, delayed orgasm on certain medications, intrusive thoughts, and fear of rejection after a history of pressure. Pick two brakes that show up most often and write one intervention for each. If conflict lingers, schedule repairs within twenty-four hours and avoid late-night confrontations in bed. If labor is uneven, reassign tasks before you try to reassign desire. If pelvic pain appears, pursue pelvic floor therapy, evaluate for vestibulodynia or endometriosis when relevant, and reorganize sex around external pleasure while treatment proceeds. If erections vary, extend warm up, engage pressure and rhythm that work reliably, use devices without apology, and coordinate with a clinician about cardiovascular and hormone health. If medication delays orgasm, schedule longer windows, use steadier patterns once close, and speak with a prescriber about adjustments.

Health integration turns sexual wellbeing from a wish into care. Make a list of clinicians you can consult: primary care, gynecology, urology, pelvic floor therapy, sex therapy when helpful. Add the scripts you plan to use at appointments so that you speak clearly under stress. I want full STI screening today because I have a new partner. Penetration hurts at the entrance and I would like an exam for vestibulodynia and a referral to pelvic floor physical therapy. My antidepressant delays orgasm and I want to discuss dose, timing, or alternatives. My erections have changed and I want a cardiovascular evaluation and a discussion of options. Bring notes about what you have tried. Bring a partner if you want support. Decline shame. Accept evidence-based care.

Ethics about pregnancy prevention deserve space even if you never plan to conceive. Contraception lowers background anxiety. Choose methods after accurate counseling. Combined hormonal methods often lighten bleeding and cramps; some users notice mood and libido shifts. Progestin-only methods fit some bodies better and avoid estrogen. Copper IUDs avoid hormones and can increase bleeding at first. Fertility awareness can work well with training and consistent application, especially when paired with barriers during uncertain days. Emergency contraception is a responsible tool, not proof of failure. If you are at risk of pregnancy and live where abortion care is uncertain, write contingency steps into your plan so that fear does not consume arousal.

Privacy and digital hygiene protect relationships and reputations. Decide how you will store explicit messages or photos if you create them. Use encrypted vaults instead of general camera rolls. Disable cloud backups for intimate media. Remove identifying objects from frames. Confirm deletion agreements with partners when relationships change. Write consent into sexting: ask before sending; check whether the other is in a safe place to receive; decline respectfully when you are not. Set boundaries around porn use that match your values and your relationship agreements. Agency is the test. If you can pause use, rotate media types, and discuss openly, the tool is serving you. If secrecy grows or variety disappears, revise.

Communication practices must be built into the plan rather than added when things go wrong. Short phrases for in-the-moment steering keep scenes on track: softer, slower, stay there, higher, lower, keep the rhythm, pause, breathe with me. A two-sentence debrief afterward consolidates learning: one thing that worked, one change for next time. A weekly ten-minute meeting outside the bedroom protects the topic from stress. Review one success, one friction point, and schedule at least one window that respects physiology. Confirm any medical or family constraints. Ask one small question that leads to an action within seven days. The brevity keeps the habit alive.

Consent deserves structure that survives arousal. Agree on how you start, what check-ins sound like, and what stop signals you will use. The traffic light format remains serviceable because it is short and clear. Pair any stop with a promised sequence: water, eye contact, calm tone, reset. Add plans for dissociation or freeze if those have appeared in the past: keep faces visible, anchor with present-tense statements, slow breathing together, end the scene without debate. Consent stored as muscle memory lowers worry for everyone involved.

Rituals turn good intentions into repeatable action. A small beginning ritual signals to the body that intimacy is about to start. You can silence notifications, set the lamp, rinse your face, choose music, and stand together for three slow breaths before touching. An ending ritual prevents the experience from evaporating into confusion or fatigue. Water, a snack, holding in a comfortable position, a warm cloth, a sentence of appreciation, a promise for the next time you will meet, these simple steps tell the nervous system to store the memory as positive and complete.

Solo practice belongs inside partnered plans because it trains attention and expands repertoire. Write how you will keep a private relationship with your own arousal: frequency that suits your season, a short room setup, a few fantasies phrased as themes you respect, toys and lubricants that work for your body, edging experiments to learn the edge between enough and too much, a three-line log to notice patterns without turning sex into data entry. Private confidence often makes partnered sex easier because you can lead and you can teach.

Partnered skill building needs its own calendar. Pick one theme per month so that learning does not disappear under the day's noise. A month can focus on longer warm up and slower transitions. Another can focus on clitoral mapping or frenulum mapping with specific feedback. Another can focus on steady rhythm once close to orgasm. Another can focus on initiation redesign, where each person practices an approach that actually fits the receiver's nervous system. Another can focus on fantasy translation into simple, consented lines spoken out loud. Routine keeps growth from depending on mood.

Design for mismatched desire with precision rather than blame. One partner may experience frequent spontaneous desire; the other may experience responsive desire that appears only after arousal begins. Accept the difference and move to logistics. Agree on windows that suit both bodies. Earlier hours often beat midnight. Allow "begin without promising a particular outcome" as a valid entry; many responsive-desire partners find that saying yes to warm up lets desire arrive later. Expand what counts so that there are more ways to say yes. Protect refusal with warmth by pairing a no with an alternate path and a specific reschedule.

Shame resilience belongs in the plan because shame silences learning. Many carry scripts that call pleasure selfish, label certain bodies unworthy, or frame desire as proof of defect. You can write accurate counters that you repeat on purpose. Pleasure inside consent and care reflects health. My body today is eligible for comfort. Boundaries protect connection. Asking teaches my partner how to love me. A sentence read before a scene can change a night because expectation drives arousal. If the old story returns in the middle, speak the counter quietly and return to sensation.

Trauma-informed steps protect nervous systems that learned to brace. Start outside the pelvis and move in slowly over weeks, not minutes. Keep faces visible if losing sight spikes fear. Limit duration at first and end while the body still feels safe. Stabilize with predictable routines and clear signals to stop. Pair intimate touch with breath you count aloud together. Practice aftercare even when the scene stays gentle. Keep a standing therapy appointment if intrusive images or avoidance persist, and coordinate care among clinicians so that messages match. Progress measured in presence rather than in intensity becomes durable progress.

Create a troubleshooting section that you can open on hard nights without insulting yourselves. When arousal will not start, check context first: fatigue, conflict, and distractions erode attention. Shorten the scene and choose closeness without a goal. When orgasm stalls, keep location, pressure, and rhythm constant once close; many people change something at the last minute and drop the wave. When erections fade, slow the pace, reduce performance language, add a toy or a sleeve, and return to pressure and rhythm that work. When penetration hurts, stop penetration and protect the association by choosing external pleasure while you seek care. When desire feels absent for weeks, scale expectations, protect connection, and bring the topic to a clinician to review medications, hormones, pain, mood, and sleep.

Learning plans keep curiosity alive. Decide which sources you will consult during the next six months. A trustworthy book, an anatomy class, a workshop on consent, a pelvic floor appointment, a podcast that respects ethics, an educator whose work matches your values. Choose one at a time. Integrate what helps. Retire what does not. Do not drown in tips. Desire does better with two changes that fit than with twenty tricks that do not.

Life transitions demand revisions. Illness changes energy, sensation, positions, and timing. Grief narrows focus and makes tenderness more important than intensity. Postpartum months require patience, lubricant, pelvic floor care, and flexible definitions of success. Menopause adjusts tissue and sleep; local estrogen and moisturizers can help tissue, earlier hours can help attention, slower pacing can help arousal. Retirement changes schedules and can change identity; routine and novelty need to be redesigned. Moves, job loss, caregiving for parents, gender transition, and repartnering all belong in the plan.

When seasons shift, make an appointment with each other to rewrite logistics and expectations.

Relationship structure shapes practice. Monogamous couples renew rather than police. A weekly desire message, a predictable intimacy window, alternating initiation, a quarterly experiment agreed upon in writing, appreciation spoken aloud, these habits keep exclusivity fertile. Nonmonogamous networks need health protocols, disclosure practices, time buffers, aftercare for everyone involved, and repair skills when jealousy or scheduling mistakes hurt. Write those systems down. Revisit them often. Care is the reputation you carry.

Digital sex deserves recap inside this plan even if you covered it earlier. Decide what kinds of porn fit your ethics and attention. Decide where you will store intimate media. Decide how you will consent to sending or receiving explicit content. Decide which creators or communities support your arousal without leaving you depleted. Decide how often devices stay out of the room where you want to touch. Protect the future version of you who will scroll back through your history and feel relief rather than dread.

Neurodivergence thrives with explicit structure. If you are autistic, write sensory preferences for light, sound, temperature, fabrics, and pressure; include a scene order you like; reduce surprises; use written agreements and visual timers. If you have ADHD, prefer earlier hours, brief focused scenes, verbal anchors that keep attention inside the body, and agreements about phones. If you live with OCD or scrupulosity, choose rituals that stabilize without escalating compulsions; start scenes with a one-minute grounding practice and end with a brief gratitude sentence; keep therapy in the loop. None of this removes passion. It creates access to it.

Disability invites creativity. Pillows can turn a bed into a stable platform. Chairs can become allies. Toys can transfer effort from small joints to larger muscles. Shorter scenes with longer aftercare can respect pain conditions. Coordinating sex with medication timing and energy peaks makes more difference than willpower ever did. Partners ask what works today and mean it. Plans that respect limits protect desire because bodies stop bracing.

Community support enlarges your capacity. List people and places that keep you brave: clinicians who treat sexual health kindly, educators who teach without shaming, friends who speak plainly, groups that normalize your questions, faith communities that center dignity and consent. You do not need a crowd. You need a few reliable sources that you trust when the internet feels loud.

Vignettes can help you see how a plan looks in real life.

Picture two parents who have been exhausted for a year. They read their compass aloud on a Sunday morning: playful, warm, honest. They move sex from 10 p.m. to Saturday afternoon during naptime. They put a lock on the bedroom door and a towel in the drawer with lube. They agree that external pleasure counts as complete twice a week and penetration will only return if comfort is consistent for a month. They start a ten-minute check-in on Sunday nights. Four weeks later both report more ease and fewer fights about rejection.

Picture a single reader with responsive desire who believed they were broken. They create a solo practice twice a week in the morning before work, dim a lamp, use a vibrator for external stimulation, practice edging, and write three lines afterward about what helped. They keep porn off the menu for a month to retrain attention with imagination and audio erotica that fits their ethics. After six weeks desire arrives faster because the body recognizes the path.

Picture a midlife couple navigating delayed orgasm from medication and inconsistent erections after prostate treatment.

They extend warm up, shift to earlier hours, keep pressure and rhythm steady once close, and bring a wand and a sleeve into partnered scenes with humor and care. They schedule pelvic floor therapy for both. They meet with clinicians to review medications. They add a rule that praise must be spoken out loud. Sex changes shape and stays central.

Picture a nonbinary reader who has avoided sex because of dysphoria. They write language for their body that lands well. They choose clothes that affirm identity and positions that keep attention on parts that feel congruent. They ask for consent scripts that include visible faces and predictable order of operations. They plan scenes that use external focus and mouth on neck and chest rather than direct genital attention until safety holds. Pleasure returns because identity is honored.

Picture a polyamorous network that decides to standardize health practices. Quarterly testing, barriers with new partners until two clean panels have passed, shared calendars that include recovery buffers after dates, agreements about disclosures, aftercare that includes messages home, and a review meeting every month. The network steadies because care is visible.

Measurement keeps hubris and despair from running the show. Count what matches your values. You might track how often you protected a window, how often you repaired within twenty-four hours, how often you spoke a desire out loud, how often sex felt comfortable in your body, how often you ended with aftercare instead of collapse. Use numbers as signals, not as grades.

Repair language belongs in the back pocket for the day you need it. The person who pushed or missed a cue says what happened, apologizes, and proposes a change. The person who was hurt names impact and requests what would restore trust. Both agree on a small plan and a review date. Brevity helps. I sped up when I felt you getting close. I am sorry. Next time I will ask whether to keep the same rhythm. I froze when your hand moved without asking. I need you to check before touching my chest. Let us try again on Sunday afternoon with more time and a pause for breath.

Put all of this onto one document and give it a home. The first page carries your compass and principles. The second page maps context and timing. The third summarizes body preferences and brakes with interventions. The fourth lists health care notes and clinician scripts. The fifth defines privacy and digital agreements. The sixth outlines rituals for beginning and ending. The seventh sets communication habits and consent signals. The eighth schedules monthly learning and practice themes. The ninth holds troubleshooting steps. The tenth records review dates and small wins. You can keep it private or share sections with a partner. You can change anything that stops serving you.

Set a start date within a week. Put a brief meeting on the calendar. Read your plan aloud. Choose one change you can make without anyone else's permission, such as moving the lamp, placing lube within reach, or setting a morning window. Choose one change that benefits from collaboration, such as a consent signal, a weekly check-in, or a medical appointment. Place the next review date before you stand up.

A plan cannot remove grief, illness, or the randomness of life. A plan can reduce avoidable obstacles, teach your body to expect kindness, and give you a method for returning to pleasure when weeks are hard. Most important, a plan keeps sex aligned with the kind of person you want to be. When your choices follow your compass, desire becomes easier to trust. It shows up more often because you have built a place for it to live.

Chapter 18
Conclusion: Sexuality as an Ongoing Practice

Every chapter in this book has been a way of saying the same thing with more detail and more care: sexual wellbeing grows when you treat it as a practice. Skills improve through repetition, bodies respond to context, desire shows up when conditions are friendly, and love becomes sturdier when people choose design over guessing. A practice does not need perfection. A practice needs attention, kindness, and the willingness to return.

Consider how most of us first learned about sex. Lessons arrived in fragments, or as warnings with missing steps, or through images that looked thrilling and felt distant from our own bodies. Very few were taught to notice breath, to name what touch actually feels like, to speak about consent in ordinary rooms, to ask for pace and pressure with the same ease used to ask for salt at dinner. The absence of those lessons did not erase the capacity for pleasure. It simply delayed fluency. You can claim fluency now. You can decide that your erotic life deserves the same steady care you offer to work you value, to friendships you protect, and to the kitchen you stock with food that suits you.

Return for a moment to the basic map. Each person carries accelerators and brakes. Accelerators respond to cues of safety, affection, time, novelty, competence, praise, privacy, and play. Brakes respond to stress, shame, unfinished fights, pain, fatigue, distraction, and fear. None of us control every cue in the world outside. All of us can shape some of them close to home.

When you choose earlier windows because late night has never been kind to you, that is practice. When you keep lube where you can reach it without breaking eye contact, that is practice. When you send a message at lunch that plants a small seed for evening, that is practice. When you repair a miss within a day and propose one change for next time, that is practice. Desire begins to trust people who behave this way.

The nervous system keeps score. Not with arithmetic, but with predictions. After enough experiences where boundaries were honored, bodies breathe before they are touched. After enough evenings where care followed intensity, bodies anticipate comfort and let go sooner. After enough scenes where specific words led to specific actions, bodies stop bracing for confusion. This is one reason communication carries such power. Words that match behavior teach the brain to lower the guard. The language here is smaller than romance often promises, and more effective. Softer. Stay there. Slower. Yes, more. Pause. Breathe with me. Those phrases are not therapy slogans. They are the handles that open doors.

Practice thrives in pairs and it thrives alone. Private erotic life has been treated as a side note for too long, as if solo touch were merely an answer to scarcity or a teenage habit to be outgrown. This book has asked you to reframe private time as a studio where you learn your instrument. When you stay with one rhythm long enough to notice the difference between enough and too much, you are training attention. When you map the border of the clitoral hood or the frenulum and memorize the angle that matters, you are writing a manual your partner will one day thank you for. When you test whether fantasy leads or follows sensation and discover that alternating works best for your mind, you are building a bridge between imagination and body. Solo practice then enriches partnered scenes because you can guide with clarity rather than with hope.

Partners who treat sex as a shared craft move through seasons with more ease. They notice the way family life narrows privacy and they plan around it. They notice the way grief reduces appetite and they choose tenderness without calling it failure. They notice the way hormones change tissue and they welcome new lubricants, new hours, and new sequences. They notice the way performance anxiety grows when novelty arrives too fast and they choose smaller experiments. The choice is not between passion and planning. The choice is between pressure and permission. Planning that honors bodies offers permission for play.

Consent remains the center. Not as a legal checkbox, not as a speech written for a class, but as a living agreement people can feel in their bodies. Consent that works in real bedrooms uses short signals, predictable pauses, and aftercare as a promise, not a maybe. Red means stop. Yellow means slow or change something specific. Green means keep going. Stop is followed by water, eye contact, calm voice, and a reset. These rituals sound simple. They undo years of ambivalence because the nervous system receives evidence that saying no does not end love, that pausing does not invite punishment, that boundaries increase connection instead of threatening it. The result is not fewer orgasms. The result is more trust.

The same consent habits carry you into edges and play. Kink and power exchange have often been described as a world apart, when the underlying skills are the same ones that make ordinary sex possible. Clear negotiation in daylight. Signals that stop the scene. Attention to breath and tone. Aftercare that respects the person who gave and the person who received. If you are curious, begin at the edges of what you already do. Let one person lead pace for fifteen minutes while the other practices following. Trade who speaks and who stays quiet. Try a steady rhythm of impact on places with muscle rather than bone and keep your check-ins simple. Praise the parts that worked. Retire the parts that did not. People who handle power with care often discover tenderness growing where tension used to live.

Digital life needs to sit beside the bed without crawling into it uninvited. Phones can introduce lovers, deliver desire in a sentence, and carry voice when distance would otherwise empty the week. Phones can also scatter attention, archive private moments in unsafe places, and inject other people's bodies into rooms where you wish to look only at the one you chose. Your practice here is agency. Decide which media support arousal without leaving you depleted. Decide how you ask consent before sending an image and how you protect images once they exist. Decide how you will store or delete when a bond changes. Decide how often your devices leave the bedroom so that your mind can rest on skin instead of on light.

Queer and trans readers have carried the cost of secrecy and scrutiny longer than most, often from childhood. The body learns to scan for danger, to plan exits, to speak softly in rooms where plain truth would invite harm. If this is your history, let the final pages name your skill and your right to joy. You have practised vigilance so well that you can now practise rest. Choose partners who affirm language for your body. Insist on consent scripts that include pronouns and parts. Design scenes that keep attention on the places that feel like home, and change the scenes when dysphoria surges. Ask for care from clinicians who know your anatomy and your identity, both. Include chosen family in the circle that keeps you brave. Pleasure belongs to you, and so does the pace that lets you receive it.

Trauma is not a disqualifier. The nervous system remembers to protect, and that memory can be honored while building new associations. Start far from the places that carried hurt. Touch shoulders and scalp and the sides of ribs. Keep faces where you can see them. Pair each transition with breath counted out loud. End while the body still feels inside tolerance. Practice aftercare even when touch remained modest. Ask for therapy when memories intrude or when avoidance steals months. Celebrate presence over intensity. That measure, sustained over time, transforms rooms.

Health is part of sex. Pelvic pain deserves evaluation and gentle therapy. Hormone changes deserve accurate counseling and tools that protect tissue. Medications that shift arousal deserve creative adjustments and conversations with prescribers who do not blush. Erection changes ask for patience, sleeves and toys, and medical screening that protects the heart as well as the penis. Lubricants belong on nightstands without apology. Dilators belong in treatment plans when entrances need to relearn ease. PDE5 inhibitors, local estrogen, pelvic floor release, sleep, grief support, and disability aids, all of these are acts of love, not signs of defeat.

Relationships need structure that fits the people inside them. Some bonds flourish within exclusivity that is renewed on purpose. Some bonds flourish within agreements that widen the field. Both require honesty, boundaries, health practices, repair, and gentleness with feelings that arrive uninvited. Jealousy offers information that can be answered with reassurance and better calendars. New relationship energy needs fences that protect a home base. Metamours are people, not puzzles to solve. Children require stability no matter what structure the adults choose. A practice approach keeps ideology out of the bedroom and puts kindness back in.

Aging does not remove erotic capacity. Bodies change, sensation shifts, patience grows, and the meaning of sex often deepens. Perimenopause invites slower pacing, more external focus, high quality lubricant, and local estrogen when appropriate. Andropause language may be imprecise, yet many men notice slower arousal and benefit from longer warm up and a broader menu. Disabled bodies and chronically ill bodies do not fall outside the circle. They teach us to design for energy, to value shorter scenes with longer aftercare, to recruit pillows and chairs and tools as allies, to ask each time what would make this day possible. There is no age at which tenderness stops working.

Culture enters the room. Faith traditions, family expectations, community norms, and laws around reproductive care and identity shape how safe a person feels while naked with someone they trust. None of us control the world. All of us can create small zones where our values set the tone. Consent, dignity, mutual care, honesty about consequences, and protection of the vulnerable are values that travel well. When these live in a house, children grow up with words that fit their bodies, adults handle differences with less panic, and sex can remain part of ordinary health rather than a secret or a performance.

The last pages of a book are a good place for instructions that sound like blessings. Keep your plan somewhere you can touch it. Read it aloud to yourself or to a partner when drift appears. Protect time with the same seriousness you reserve for appointments that pay the bills. Speak appreciation out loud in complete sentences and do it often enough that the person you love could imitate your voice. Decline with warmth and offer alternate paths so that no turns into care rather than into distance. Ask for what you want in language that a body can follow. Listen until your partner's shoulders drop. Repair quickly and specifically. Store aftercare as a habit, not as a treat. Remember that fun is a kind of medicine.

Rituals help the mind remember what the heart already knows. Begin with three breaths together before any scene, a tiny ceremony that tells the room who you are to each other. End with water, a simple snack, a warm cloth, a word of thanks, and a promise about next time. Keep one song that belongs to sex only, and let it serve as an entrance cue whenever you press play. Write one sentence each week that names something you want to repeat. Put a lock on the door and call it care. Leave your phone outside sometimes and call that care too.

There are readers who will close this book during a difficult season. Illness has narrowed options. Work has stolen attention. Grief has dampened appetite. Conflict has left a mark that still stings. If this is where you find yourself, stay gentle. The project is not to force a body to perform. The project is to keep a thread in your hand so that you can find your way back when the road brightens. Ten minutes of sensual attention without a goal, a bath with slow breath, a message sent or received that says I want you in the body you have today, a promise to ask your clinician one clear question, these are practice steps. They count.

There are readers who will close this book buzzing with possibility. New habits have already changed nights. Conversations feel less dangerous. A toy waits in the drawer. A playlist sits ready. A check-in lives on the calendar. If this is where you find yourself, do not rush to collect scenes. Collect evidence of steadiness. Keep experiments small enough to succeed. Praise each other out loud. Let your bodies learn that pleasure is available more often than you were taught to expect.

A final story, offered in pieces you can carry. Two people sit at a table on a Sunday afternoon. They pour tea. They read the notes they made last month about what worked. One says that earlier hours helped, and that praise after sex changed something quiet inside. The other says that the new consent signal felt easy to use and that the shower together on Thursday mattered more than they expected. They look at the week ahead and circle one hour in pencil. They write a plan in ten words. Music. Kissing. Shower. External focus. Ask before chest. Water. Hold. They place lube where hands can find it. They turn off notifications and put the phones face down in another room. When the hour arrives, neither is surprised by what happens next. They know how to begin. They know how to steer. They know how to stop and how to care. Nothing cinematic occurs. Everything essential does. The nervous systems talk to each other. The room learns another story about safety. Desire arrives as a guest who recognizes the address.

Now imagine the same practice held by one person on a morning where solitude is the gift. A lamp is dim. A towel waits. A glass of water sits within reach. The person opens a small notebook, reads a line about a theme that works for them, and closes their eyes. Breath slows. The first touch remains wide and gentle. Minutes pass. Edges appear and soften. When the session ends, three sentences go on the page. What helped. What interfered. What to try next time. The entry takes less than a minute. The body carries the rest all day.

Books end. Practices continue. You will forget and remember and forget again. You will enter seasons where sex feels like home and seasons where sex feels like a language you once spoke. Keep the tools nearby. Keep kindness nearby. Keep curiosity nearby. The body you live in today is eligible for comfort and for joy. The person you love is eligible for clarity and for care. The future you is eligible for stories that feel good to remember.

If a single line from these pages is worth tucking into your pocket, let it be this one. Pleasure grows where people are safe, seen, and spoken to with care. Give that to yourself. Give that to your partners. Give that to the communities you touch. When you do, sexuality stops acting like a test and starts behaving like a practice that keeps you connected to your body, to your values, and to the people who matter to you. That practice can last a lifetime.

Bonus Chapter
Breath, Pelvic Floor, and the Mechanics of Arousal

Pleasure rides on physiology. You can adore your partner, have rich fantasy, feel emotionally safe, and still struggle if breath is shallow, pelvic muscles hold tension, or nerves fire under stress chemistry. This chapter treats the body as an instrument you can tune. When breath lengthens, muscles coordinate, and blood flow meets sensation, arousal becomes easier to access and easier to repeat.

Start with breath because it sets the tone for the whole nervous system. Inhalation gears attention toward action. Exhalation gears attention toward rest and digestion. Erotic states ask for both. A useful baseline involves breathing through the nose when possible, letting the ribs move outward and the belly move forward, then exhaling until the lower ribs settle back toward center. That long exhale recruits the branch of the nervous system that lets arousal build without tipping into vigilance. Many people think they should breathe faster as sensation rises. Many bodies prefer slower, deeper breaths that keep oxygen steady and signal safety. Try a six-count inhale, hold for one beat, then an eight-count exhale, repeated for a minute before touch begins. You are not doing yoga class. You are bringing the accelerator online while letting the brakes relax.

Coordination between breath and pelvic floor matters more than most were taught. The pelvic floor is a group of muscles arranged like a hammock between the pubic bone and the tailbone. In a calm pattern these muscles lengthen slightly on inhalation and gather gently on exhalation. Stress flips the sequence. Many people clench on inhale, which raises pressure, restricts blood flow, and makes penetration or orgasm feel elusive or irritable. Rehearsal corrects this quietly. Lie on your back with knees bent, one hand on your lower ribs and one near your pubic bone. Inhale and imagine the hammock lowering a small amount. Exhale and imagine it lifting gently. The movement is subtle. The effect shows up later as comfort.

Release comes before strength for a lot of readers. Kegels became a cultural shorthand and left out half of the story. Contracting a muscle that already lives clenched increases discomfort. A more balanced practice begins with down-training. Long exhales, jaw and tongue relaxed, hips supported by pillows, and targeted stretches like child's pose, happy baby, or a figure-four glute stretch help lengthen a guarded floor. Add a few slow squats if your joints allow, focusing on ease at the bottom rather than on depth. Once length returns, strength work helps with orgasm intensity and continence. Three-second gentle contractions followed by six-second releases, for a set of eight to ten, performed two or three times a day, are enough for most. If pain, urgency, or burning accompany any of this, a pelvic floor therapist becomes your next partner.

Blood flow drives arousal, so circulation deserves attention. Warmth increases vascular responsiveness. A shower, a heated blanket, or even socks matters more than romance novels admit. Movement earlier in the day helps too. A brisk walk or light strength work sends blood to the pelvis later with less effort. Hydration supports lubrication and semen volume. Alcohol blunts sensitivity, shortens plateau phases, and increases the chance of pain the next day. Caffeine late in the day shortens patience at night. This is not a diet lecture. This is logistics for a system that wants clear signals.

Anatomy needs direct practice. For vulva owners, indirect touch first often transforms later intensity. The outer labia enjoy broad, firm pressure. The inner labia respond to glide and warmth. The clitoral hood covers the glans; rolling or circling the hood often beats direct contact at the start. Once arousal rises, steady pressure on the glans or along the hood's edge, kept consistent for longer than you think, helps the body crest. Rhythm changes early wake attention. Repetition late lets orgasm assemble. For penis owners, the frenulum and the underside near the base of the glans carry dense sensation. A grip that includes the perineum or that anchors at the base reduces overstimulation at the tip. Many partners increase speed at the moment before release. Many bodies prefer the same stroke, same squeeze, and same pace for the final seconds. When in doubt, stay until asked to change.

Orgasm timing often improves when pelvic floor and breath work together. As intensity rises, many people hold breath, tighten jaw, and clench the floor without noticing. That trio can stall climax. A simple correction involves a single cue. Keep exhaling. The sound can be quiet. The effect is real. Exhalation softens the floor just enough to let waves move instead of rebound. If release arrives too quickly and you want delay, switch to shallower exhales for a few breaths while keeping touch steady, then return to the longer pattern. Edging practices become easier when breath leads and muscles follow.

Pain deserves precise routes to relief. Burning at the vaginal entrance often points toward vestibulodynia, hormonal thinning, dermatitis, or floor hypertonicity. Lubricant helps. So does local estrogen for many in perimenopause or postpartum. So does therapy that teaches relaxation and manual release. Deep ache with certain angles suggests cervical contact. Positions that let the receiver control depth, such as being on top or side lying, protect comfort. Sharp pain in the penis with erection merits medical evaluation for curvature or plaques. Stinging with ejaculation invites a check for prostatitis. The rule that protects sex applies again. Comfort first, novelty later.

Sensory load can make or break a night. Light that flatters skin and reduces visual clutter changes how exposed people feel. Sound that blends into the room masks partner noise without drowning it. Fabrics that do not scratch or trap heat reduce distraction. Scents that belong to you two, not to the last guest in this hotel room, set a cue that triggers memory on future nights. Small sensorial edits often solve problems that looked like mismatched desire.

Neurodivergent readers benefit from visible structure. A card at the bedside with scene order removes guesswork. The card might read: three breaths together, shoulders and back for five minutes, external focus for ten, check-in, option to continue or end with holding and water. Eye contact can be intense near orgasm for autistic partners; agree in advance whether to meet eyes or to look away without meaning disconnection. ADHD attention drifts when scenes run long without anchors; agree on simple phrases like stay here or keep the pace that pull mind back to body.

Gender-affirming care intersects with mechanics. Testosterone enlarges the clitoris and changes lubrication patterns; pressure preferences may shift toward firmer touch and different angles. Estrogen reduces spontaneous erections and increases breast sensitivity; arousal benefits from longer warm up and direct attention to the chest. Postoperative anatomy has unique needs. A neovagina requires lubrication and dilation schedules tailored by the surgeon; a partner's patience becomes part of medical care. Phalloplasty and metoidioplasty change nerve maps; exploration writes a new manual rather than proving loss.

Devices deserve a place near the bed without embarrassment. External vibrators help clitoral orgasms and can travel across bodies during partnered sex. Wands overpower numb days and can be softened with towels. Sleeves reduce grip fatigue and make rhythm easier to maintain. Plugs with flared bases teach the floor to receive fullness gently. Vacuum tools can support erections as part of therapy, with or without rings, and should be introduced with humor and planfulness rather than as a last resort. Tools expand options. They do not replace intimacy.

Aftercare remains physiology, not only kindness. A face cloth warms skin. Water restores. A snack steadies blood sugar. A minute of stillness lowers heart rate. A sentence about what worked primes the next time. Many bodies enter a calm state after intense arousal. Others feel tender. Neither state requires analysis. Both benefit from a predictable close.

Keep practice honest by measuring what matters. Comfort during penetration counts more than frequency. Ability to ask in one sentence for a change counts more than endurance. Reduced vigilance counts more than a new position. Breath that stays steady at the moment you usually rush counts more than any trick. When you track these factors, you will see progress even in hard weeks, which keeps motivation alive.

Pleasure is teachable when mechanics support it. You are not chasing magic. You are adjusting inputs until the system behaves the way it was designed to behave. Breath first. Floor next. Blood flow, warmth, rhythm, and words that a body can follow. Repeat often enough to write new predictions. Then enjoy how desire arrives with less effort.

www.ingramcontent.com/pod-product-compliance
Lightning Source LLC
Chambersburg PA
CBHW050653270326
41927CB00012B/3007